Eat to latch

100 Delicious Recipes for Breastfeeding moms to support your journey

Diane Mcwells

Dedication

To all mothers around the world,

This book is dedicated to you—the nurturing hearts, the tireless caregivers, and the fearless warriors. You are the epitome of love, strength, and resilience. Your unwavering commitment to your little ones is an inspiration to us all.

In every corner of the globe, you embark on the incredible journey of motherhood, facing challenges, celebrating milestones, and embracing the joys that come with nurturing a new life. Your unwavering dedication to providing the best for your child is unparalleled.

Through sleepless nights and endless feedings, you hold your baby close, offering comfort, nourishment, and the warmth of your embrace. You navigate the intricacies of breastfeeding, selflessly giving of yourself to create a bond that transcends words.

Your love knows no boundaries, your sacrifices go unnoticed, and your strength knows no limits. This dedication is a small token of gratitude for the love, care, and endless support you pour into your little ones every single day.

May this book serve as a guiding light, a source of knowledge, and a beacon of empowerment as you embark on your breastfeeding journey. May it provide the reassurance and wisdom you seek, and may it remind you that you are not alone.

To all the mothers around the world, this book is for you. May you find solace, inspiration, and valuable insights within its pages. May it empower you to embrace the bond of breastfeeding and embark on a remarkable chapter of motherhood.

With deep admiration and respect,

[Diane Mcwells]

Table of Contents:

Chapter 7: Quick and Easy Meals for Busy Moms 111

Introduction

Embracing the Journey of Breastfeeding

Welcome to "Eat to Latch: 100 Delicious Recipes for Breastfeeding Moms to Support Your Journey." Congratulations on embarking on the incredible journey of breastfeeding! This book is designed to be your trusted companion, offering a collection of mouthwatering recipes and valuable insights to nourish and empower you on this special path.

Breastfeeding is a remarkable bonding experience between you and your little one, and proper nutrition plays a vital role in ensuring the health and well-being of both of you. In "Eat to Latch," we have curated a diverse range of recipes that are not only delicious but also thoughtfully crafted to support your breastfeeding journey.

Our goal is to provide you with a comprehensive resource that not only satisfies your cravings but also fuels your body with essential nutrients. We understand that as a breastfeeding mom, you have unique nutritional needs. That's why we've carefully selected ingredients that are known to boost milk supply, enhance milk quality, and support your postpartum recovery.

But "Eat to Latch" goes beyond just recipes. We delve into the science behind breastfeeding nutrition, helping you understand the key nutrients your body needs and how they contribute to your milk production and overall well-being. We also explore the importance of self-care, mindful eating practices, and finding balance in your busy life as a new mom.

Whether you're seeking quick and easy meals for busy days, nourishing dinners for the whole family, or satisfying snacks to keep your energy levels up, "Eat to Latch" has you covered. Each recipe is accompanied by clear instructions, helpful tips, and variations to accommodate different dietary preferences, ensuring that everyone can enjoy these culinary delights.

We want you to embrace this journey with confidence, knowing that you have the knowledge and support to make the most of your breastfeeding experience. Let "Eat to Latch" be your go-to resource, guiding you towards a nourishing and joyful breastfeeding journey.

Get ready to embark on a delicious adventure that celebrates the power of food, the bond between mother and child, and the incredible journey of breastfeeding. "Eat to Latch" is here to support and inspire you every step of the way. Let's dive in and create a nourishing and unforgettable breastfeeding experience together.

Chapter 1: The Power of Nutrition for Breastfeeding Moms

-Understanding the Nutritional Needs of Breastfeeding Moms

Breastfeeding is a remarkable journey that nourishes the bond between a mother and her baby. It is a time of immense physical and emotional changes, and proper nutrition plays a pivotal role in supporting both the mother's well-being and the growth and development of the little one. In Chapter 1 of the "Eat to Latch" cookbook, we delve into the topic of understanding the nutritional needs of breastfeeding moms, equipping them with essential knowledge to make informed choices about their diet.

One of the first key aspects we explore is the increased demand that breastfeeding places on a mother's body. Producing breast milk requires additional energy and nutrients, making it crucial for moms to prioritize their nutritional intake. Proteins, for example, play a vital role in milk production and are essential for the growth and repair of body tissues. Lean meats, poultry, fish, legumes, and dairy products are excellent sources of protein that can be incorporated into a breastfeeding mom's diet.

Carbohydrates, another essential nutrient, provide the energy necessary for both the mother and baby. Whole grains, fruits, and vegetables are excellent sources of complex carbohydrates that offer sustained energy. Additionally, healthy fats, such as those found in avocados, nuts, and olive oil, are important for brain development in infants and provide energy for the mother.

Vitamins and minerals are also crucial for breastfeeding moms. Calcium, for instance, supports bone health for both the mother and the baby. Dark leafy greens, dairy products, and fortified plant-based milks are excellent sources of calcium. Iron is another essential nutrient as breastfeeding can deplete iron stores in the mother's body. Lean red meats, poultry, fish, beans, and fortified cereals are iron-rich foods that can help replenish these stores.

In addition to understanding the specific nutrients needed, it is equally important to focus on maintaining a well-balanced and diverse diet. By "eating the rainbow," breastfeeding moms can ensure they consume a variety of fruits and vegetables, which provide a range of vitamins, minerals, and antioxidants necessary for optimal health. By incorporating a wide array of colors into their meals, moms can enhance the nutritional quality of their breast milk, providing their babies with a broad spectrum of nutrients.

Hydration is another vital aspect that breastfeeding moms must pay attention to. Breast milk is composed mostly of water, so staying adequately hydrated is essential for maintaining a healthy milk supply. Drinking water throughout the day, consuming hydrating foods like fruits and vegetables, and paying attention to thirst cues are all important strategies for maintaining proper hydration.

While a nutritious diet is the foundation, some breastfeeding moms may also benefit from supplements. Vitamin D, for example, is important for bone health and can be obtained through sunlight exposure or supplements. Omega-3 fatty acids, found in fish and certain plant-based sources like flaxseeds, can support brain development. Iron supplementation may be necessary for some women if their levels are found to be low. It is always advisable to consult healthcare professionals to determine individual supplement needs.

Understanding the nutritional needs of breastfeeding moms is vital for both their own health and the well-being of their babies. By embracing this knowledge and making informed dietary choices, moms can provide their bodies with the necessary fuel to support optimal milk production and ensure the overall vitality of themselves and their little ones. Chapter 1 of the "Eat to Latch" cookbook serves as an invaluable resource, empowering breastfeeding moms to nourish themselves and their babies through the power of nutrition.

- Key Nutrients for Boosting Milk Supply

This chapter explores the issue of essential foods for increasing milk production. Understanding the function of certain nutrients helps maintain and improve milk supply, which is a major issue for many nursing mothers.

Protein is a crucial component for encouraging milk production. Inadequate protein consumption has the potential to affect milk production since protein supplies the essential building blocks for the formation of breast milk. A nursing mother may assist guarantee an appropriate protein intake by including lean meats, poultry, fish, eggs, dairy products, legumes, and plant-based protein sources like tofu and tempeh in her diet.

Iron is yet another crucial component for milk production. Low milk production, exhaustion, and lower energy levels in nursing mothers may all be caused by an iron deficiency. Lean red meats, chicken, fish, fortified cereals, beans, lentils, and dark leafy greens are among iron-rich foods that may help raise iron levels and promote healthy milk supply.

Omega-3 fatty acids are especially advantageous for nursing mothers since they help stimulate milk production and provide vital nutrients for the growing baby's brain. Omega-3 fatty acids are abundant in fatty fish like salmon and sardines as well as plant-based foods like chia seeds, flaxseeds, and walnuts.

Another essential mineral for nursing mothers is calcium since it helps with milk production and bone health. Dark leafy greens like kale and spinach, fortified plant-based milks, dairy products, and calcium-enriched foods are all excellent sources of calcium that nursing mothers may include in their diets.

Additionally, sustaining milk production depends on staying hydrated. Drinking water often throughout the day, eating hydrating meals like fruits and vegetables, and paying attention to thirst signals may all help milk production function at its best.

Despite the fact that these nutrients are crucial for milk production, it's vital to remember that nursing is a supply and demand process. More cues are delivered to the body to create milk the more often and successfully a woman pumps or a baby breastfeed. The production of milk is aided by proper nutrition, but it is crucial to discuss any worries about a low milk supply with a healthcare provider who can provide advice and assistance.

Breastfeeding mothers may use Chapter 1 of the "Eat to Latch" cookbook as a helpful resource for learning and consuming crucial foods that can increase milk production. Moms may promote their milk production and provide their kids the nutrition they need by including meals high in protein, iron, omega-3 fatty acids, calcium, and keeping hydrated.

- Foods to Enhance Milk Quality

While breast milk naturally gives infants the best nourishment possible, certain meals may improve the quality of that nutrition and provide the baby extra advantages for their growth and development.

Healthy fat-rich diets are one kind of food that may improve the quality of milk. Consuming foods rich in healthy fats, including salmon, avocados, almonds, and seeds, may help boost the amount of good fats, such omega-3 fatty acids, in breast milk. The growth of the baby's brain and nervous system depends heavily on these lipids. These foods may help nursing mothers produce more milk with greater concentrations of these vital fats by being included in their diet.

Foods high in antioxidants are essential for improving milk quality. Antioxidants support general health by defending the body's cells from the harm caused by free radicals. Antioxidants are abundant in colorful fruits and vegetables including bell peppers, citrus fruits, berries, and leafy greens. Breastfeeding mothers may raise the antioxidant content of their breast milk and provide their infants extra immune-boosting advantages by consuming a range of these colorful foods in their diet.

A further factor in improved milk quality is ingesting meals high in vitamins and minerals. The growth of the unborn child depends on folate, which is abundant in dark leafy greens like spinach and kale. Strawberries and citrus fruits both include vitamin C, which helps the body absorb iron from plant-based meals. Including more nutrient-dense foods in your diet, such as whole grains, lean proteins, dairy products, and fortified plant-based milks, will help you make sure you're getting enough vitamins and minerals.

Keeping hydrated is a further consideration for improving milk quality. Water consumption throughout the day must be enough to sustain optimum milk production and ensure that breast milk is well hydrated. Dehydration and a reduction in milk production are further problems that may be avoided with adequate hydration. Melons, cucumbers, and soups are examples of foods high in water that nursing mothers may include in their meals to help them stay hydrated.

While including these items in a nursing mother's diet might improve the quality of breast milk, a well-balanced and diverse diet is essential overall. Breastfeeding mothers may maximize the nutritional content of their breast milk and provide their newborns the greatest nutrition possible by eating a variety of nutrient-dense meals and keeping hydrated.

Chapter 2: Breakfasts to Fuel Your Day

- Energizing Smoothie Bowls

Smoothie bowls have become a popular choice for breakfast, and with good reason. They offer a refreshing and nutritious way to start your day, providing a burst of energy and a wealth of essential nutrients. In this chapter of the "Eat to Latch" cookbook, we dive into the world of energizing smoothie bowls, offering a variety of recipes to fuel your mornings.

These delightful bowls are not only visually appealing but also packed with goodness. They begin with a base of frozen fruits, such as luscious berries, ripe bananas, or tropical mangoes. These fruits not only provide natural sweetness but also offer a range of antioxidants that support overall health and well-being.

To boost the nutritional content, leafy greens like spinach or kale can be added to the mix. These vibrant greens are rich in vitamins, minerals, and fiber, making them an excellent addition to any smoothie bowl.

For a protein boost, consider incorporating ingredients such as Greek yogurt, plant-based protein powders, or a dollop of nut butter. Protein is essential for tissue repair and maintenance, keeping you feeling full and satisfied throughout the morning.

Healthy fats are another key component of an energizing smoothie bowl. Avocado, chia seeds, flaxseeds, or a drizzle of nut butter can provide nourishing fats that contribute to a feeling of satiety and provide a source of sustainable energy.

Once the smoothie base is blended to perfection, it's time for the fun part - toppings! Fresh fruits like sliced bananas, juicy berries, or tangy kiwi add bursts of flavor and vibrant colors. Crunchy toppings such as granola, chopped nuts, or toasted coconut flakes provide texture and an enjoyable contrast to the creamy base. For an extra boost of nutrients, consider sprinkling superfoods like goji berries, cacao nibs, or hemp seeds.

The beauty of smoothie bowls lies in their versatility. The "Eat to Latch" cookbook offers a range of recipes to suit different tastes and preferences. Whether you prefer a tropical twist with pineapple and coconut or a classic combination of berries and almond butter, there is a smoothie bowl recipe to satisfy every palate.

By starting your day with an energizing smoothie bowl, you're not only treating yourself to a delicious breakfast but also nourishing your body and providing it with the fuel it needs. These bowls are specifically designed to support your energy levels, promote overall well-being, and enhance the nutritional quality of your breast milk.

Get ready to indulge in the delightful world of energizing smoothie bowls with the "Eat to Latch" cookbook. These recipes will inspire you to create colorful and nutritious breakfasts that will leave you feeling energized, satisfied, and ready to embrace the day ahead.

Energizing smoothie bowl along with their ingredients, instructions, and approximate prep time:

1. Berry Burst Smoothie Bowl:

- **Ingredients:**
  - 1 cup frozen mixed berries
  - 1 cup fresh spinach
  - ½ cup Greek yogurt
  - ½ cup almond milk
  - 1 tablespoon chia seeds
- Toppings:
  - Fresh berries
  - Granola
  - Sliced almonds
- **Instructions**:
  1. In a blender, combine the frozen mixed berries, spinach, Greek yogurt, almond milk, and chia seeds.
  2. Blend until smooth and creamy.
  3. Pour the smoothie into a bowl.
  4. Top with fresh berries, granola, and sliced almonds.
- **Prep Time: 5 minutes**

2. Tropical Paradise Smoothie Bowl:

- **Ingredients**:
  - 1 cup frozen mango chunks
  - ½ cup pineapple chunks
  - ½ cup coconut milk
  - 1 cup spinach
  - 1 ripe banana
- **Toppings**:
  - Sliced banana
  - Toasted coconut flakes
  - Chopped macadamia nuts
- **Instructions**:
  1. In a blender, combine the frozen mango chunks, pineapple chunks, coconut milk, spinach, and ripe banana.
  2. Blend until smooth and creamy.
  3. Transfer the smoothie to a bowl.
  4. Top with sliced banana, toasted coconut flakes, and chopped macadamia nuts.
  - Prep Time: 5 minutes

3. Green Goddess Smoothie Bowl:

- **Ingredients**:
  - 2 cups fresh spinach
  - 1 ripe banana
  - 2 tablespoons almond butter

  - 1 cup almond milk
  - 1 tablespoon hemp seeds
- **Toppings**:
  - Kiwi slices
  - Fresh berries
  - Pumpkin seeds
- **Instructions**:
  1. In a blender, combine the fresh spinach, ripe banana, almond butter, almond milk, and hemp seeds.
  2. Blend until smooth and creamy.
  3. Pour the smoothie into a bowl.
  4. Top with kiwi slices, fresh berries, and pumpkin seeds.
  - **Prep Time: 5 minutes**

4. Peanut Butter Power Smoothie Bowl:

- **Ingredients**:
  - 2 frozen bananas
  - ½ cup Greek yogurt
  - 2 tablespoons peanut butter
  - 1 cup almond milk
  - 1 tablespoon cocoa powder
- **Toppings:**
  - Sliced banana
  - Granola
  - Drizzle of peanut butter
- **Instructions**:
  1. In a blender, combine the frozen bananas, Greek yogurt, peanut butter, almond milk, and cocoa powder.

2. Blend until smooth and creamy.

3. Transfer the smoothie to a bowl.

4. Top with sliced banana, granola, and a drizzle of peanut butter.

- **Prep Time: 5 minutes**

Enjoy these energizing smoothie bowl recipes to kick-start your day with a delicious and nutritious breakfast!

- Protein-Packed Pancakes

Protein-packed pancakes are a delicious and nutritious way to fuel your morning. This recipe combines whole wheat flour, protein powder, and other wholesome ingredients to create fluffy and satisfying pancakes. These pancakes are not only a treat for your taste buds but also provide the added benefit of protein to support your energy levels and keep you feeling full longer. Let's dive into the recipe and start flipping some delicious pancakes!

Protein-Packed Pancakes

Here's a recipe for protein-packed pancakes that will provide you with a satisfying and nutritious breakfast:

- **Ingredients:**
  - 1 cup whole wheat flour

- 1 scoop of your favorite protein powder (vanilla or unflavored)
- 1 teaspoon baking powder
- 1/2 teaspoon cinnamon
- 1 ripe banana, mashed
- 1 cup milk of your choice (dairy or plant-based)
- 1 tablespoon honey or maple syrup
- 1 teaspoon vanilla extract
- 1 tablespoon coconut oil or cooking spray for greasing the pan

- Instructions:

1. In a large mixing bowl, combine the whole wheat flour, protein powder, baking powder, and cinnamon.

2. In a separate bowl, mix together the mashed banana, milk, honey or maple syrup, and vanilla extract.

3. Pour the wet ingredients into the dry ingredients and stir until well combined. The batter should be thick but pourable. If needed, you can add a little more milk to adjust the consistency.

4. Heat a non-stick skillet or griddle over medium heat and grease it with coconut oil or cooking spray.

5. Pour about 1/4 cup of batter onto the heated skillet for each pancake. Cook until bubbles form on the surface, then flip and cook for another 1-2 minutes until golden brown.

6. Repeat the process with the remaining batter.

7. Serve the protein-packed pancakes warm and enjoy them as is or topped with your favorite toppings such as fresh berries, sliced banana, nut butter, or a drizzle of honey.

These protein-packed pancakes are not only delicious but also provide an excellent source of energy and nutrients to start your day off right. Enjoy the fluffy goodness and savor the nutritious benefits of this wholesome breakfast option.

-Wholesome Overnight Oats

Prepare a nutritious and delicious breakfast in advance with this recipe for wholesome overnight oats. It's a convenient and customizable option that will keep you fueled and satisfied throughout the morning.

- **Ingredients:**
  - 1/2 cup rolled oats
  - 1/2 cup milk of your choice (dairy or plant-based)
  - 1/2 cup Greek yogurt
  - 1 tablespoon chia seeds
  - 1 tablespoon honey or maple syrup (optional)
  - 1/2 teaspoon vanilla extract
  - Toppings of your choice: fresh berries, sliced bananas, chopped nuts, or a sprinkle of cinnamon

- **Instructions:**

1. In a jar or container, combine the rolled oats, milk, Greek yogurt, chia seeds, honey or maple syrup (if desired), and vanilla extract.

2. Stir well to ensure all the ingredients are thoroughly mixed.

3. Cover the jar or container and place it in the refrigerator overnight or for at least 4-6 hours to allow the oats to soften and absorb the flavors.

4. In the morning, give the oats a good stir and add more milk if needed to reach your desired consistency.

5. Top with your favorite toppings such as fresh berries, sliced bananas, chopped nuts, or a sprinkle of cinnamon.

6. Enjoy the wholesome overnight oats straight from the refrigerator or let them sit at room temperature for a few minutes if you prefer them slightly less chilled.

Overnight oats are a fantastic option for busy breastfeeding moms as they can be prepared ahead of time and customized to your taste preferences. They provide a balanced combination of whole grains, protein from Greek yogurt, healthy fats from chia seeds, and natural sweetness from the toppings. Feel free to experiment with different flavors and combinations to keep your breakfasts exciting and nutritious.

- Nutrient-Rich Egg Dishes

Eggs are a great source of important nutrients, making them a great option for a breakfast that is nutrient-dense. This section offers a variety of egg recipes that are nutrient-dense and high in protein, vitamins, and minerals to promote your general health. Let's investigate these healthful and tasty meals!

1. Veggie omelet

Ingredients include
 -two eggs.
 - 1/4 cup chopped, any-color bell peppers
 - One-fourth cup diced onions
 - 1/4 cup finely chopped spinach - 1 tablespoon extra virgin olive oil - salt and pepper to taste

- Requirements:
 1. In a basin, beat the eggs well.
 2. In a pan over medium heat, warm the olive oil.
 3. Add the diced onions and bell peppers to the pan and cook for 2 to 3 minutes, or until the vegetables begin to soften.
 4. Stir in the chopped spinach and cook for an additional one to two minutes, or until wilted.

5. Add salt and pepper to the beaten eggs before pouring them into the skillet.

6. Continue whisking the eggs until they are thoroughly cooked and scrambled.

7. Present the hot vegetable scramble and savor it!

10 minutes for preparation
Time to Cook: 5-7 minutes

2. Omelet with spinach and mushrooms

- ingredients:
 - 3 eggs
 - 1/4 cup sliced mushrooms - 1/2 cup chopped spinach
 2-tablespoons of diced onions
 - A dash of salt and pepper - A tablespoon of butter or frying oil

- Directions:
1. Beat the eggs in a bowl until fully combined.

2. In a non-stick skillet, heat butter or cooking oil over medium heat.

3. Add the sliced mushrooms and chopped onions to the pan and cook for 2 to 3 minutes, or until the mushrooms are beginning to soften.

4. Stir in the chopped spinach and cook for an additional one to two minutes, or until wilted.

5. Pour the beaten eggs on top of the skillet's veggies.

6. Add salt and pepper to taste.

7. Cook until the bottom is set, about 2-3 minutes.

8. To make a half-moon shape, carefully turn one side of the omelet over the other.

9. Continue cooking for a further 1-2 minutes or until the eggs are done.

10. Present the warm spinach and mushroom omelet and enjoy it!

10 minutes for preparation
Time to Cook: 5-7 minutes

These nutrient-dense egg recipes provide a balanced and delicious alternative for breakfast. Because of their adaptability, you may personalize them by adding your preferred veggies and flavors. Enjoy the benefits of eggs and the nutrition they provide while you nurse.

Chapter 3: Nourishing Lunches for Sustained Energy

- Vibrant Salad Creations

A feature of this chapter is a range of colorful salad combinations that are not only aesthetically pleasing but also filling. These salads are brimming with flavorful, colorful, and fresh ingredients. Let's look at a few dishes to get ideas for your lunches!

1. A Mediterranean quinoa salad

Ingredients:
  1 cup of cooked quinoa and 1 cup of chopped cucumbers.
  - 1 cup halved cherry tomatoes
  - A cup of finely chopped Kalamata olives
  - 1 tablespoon of lemon juice, 1/4 cup of crumbled feta cheese, 1/4 cup of fresh parsley, and 2 teaspoons of extra-virgin olive oil
  - To taste, salt and pepper

- **Requirements**:

1. Place the cooked quinoa, chopped feta cheese, sliced cucumbers, cherry tomatoes, Kalamata olives, and parsley in a large bowl.

2. To create the dressing, combine the olive oil, lemon juice, salt, and pepper in a small bowl.

3. After adding the dressing to the salad components, gently mix everything to combine.

4. Present the quinoa salad with Mediterranean flavors cold or at room temperature.

15 minutes for preparation

2. Salad made with Asian sesame chicken

Ingredients:

-2 cups cooked chicken that has been shredded; 4 cups mixed salad greens.

- One cup of grated carrots

- 1 cup of sliced, any-color bell peppers

- 1/2 cup fresh cilantro, chopped; - 1/4 cup green onions, chopped

Sesame seeds, 2 teaspoons

- Two teaspoons of low-sodium soy sauce

- 1 teaspoon sesame oil, 1 teaspoon honey, and 1 tablespoon rice vinegar

- **Requirements:**

1. Place the shredded chicken, mixed salad greens, carrots, bell pepper slices, cilantro, green onions, and sesame seeds in a big bowl.

2. To create the dressing, combine the soy sauce, rice vinegar, honey, and sesame oil in a small dish.

3. Pour the salad dressing over the contents and gently toss to mix.

4. Immediately serve the Asian sesame chicken salad.

10 minutes for preparation

These colorful salad combinations provide an inviting medley of tastes, textures, and hues. They are not only filling, but they also provide a tasty and energizing lunch alternative. You are welcome to add other veggies, meats, or dressings to these salads to suit your tastes. Take advantage of these colorful salads as part of your healthy lunch routine!

- Hearty Grain Bowls

Let us explore nourishing lunches that provide sustained energy throughout the day. One of the highlights of this chapter is the inclusion of hearty grain bowls. These bowls are packed with wholesome grains, a variety of vegetables, proteins, and flavorful dressings, creating a satisfying and nutritious meal. Let's dive into a couple of delicious grain bowl recipes to elevate your lunchtime experience!

1. Southwest Quinoa Bowl

- Ingredients:
  - 1 cup cooked quinoa
  - 1 cup black beans, drained and rinsed
  - 1 cup corn kernels (fresh or frozen)
  - 1 cup diced tomatoes
  - 1/2 cup diced red bell peppers
  - 1/4 cup chopped fresh cilantro
  - 2 tablespoons lime juice
  - 2 tablespoons olive oil
  - 1 teaspoon ground cumin
  - Salt and pepper to taste
  - Optional toppings: avocado slices, Greek yogurt, sliced jalapenos

- Instructions:
1. In a large bowl, combine the cooked quinoa, black beans, corn kernels, diced tomatoes, diced red bell peppers, and chopped cilantro.
2. In a small bowl, whisk together the lime juice, olive oil, ground cumin, salt, and pepper to create the dressing.
3. Pour the dressing over the quinoa mixture and toss gently to coat.

4. Divide the mixture into serving bowls and top with optional toppings if desired.

5. Serve the Southwest quinoa bowl and enjoy!

Prep Time: 15 minutes

2. Mediterranean Falafel Bowl

- **Ingredients:**
  - 1 cup cooked quinoa
  - 4-6 falafel balls, cooked and sliced
  - 1 cup chopped cucumbers
  - 1 cup diced tomatoes
  - 1/2 cup diced red onions
  - 1/4 cup chopped Kalamata olives
  - 1/4 cup crumbled feta cheese
  - 2 tablespoons lemon juice
  - 2 tablespoons extra-virgin olive oil
  - 1 teaspoon dried oregano
  - Salt and pepper to taste

- **Instructions**:
   1. In a large bowl, combine the cooked quinoa, sliced falafel balls, chopped cucumbers, diced tomatoes, diced red onions, chopped Kalamata olives, and crumbled feta cheese.

   2. In a small bowl, whisk together the lemon juice, olive oil, dried oregano, salt, and pepper to create the dressing.

3. Drizzle the dressing over the grain bowl ingredients and toss gently to combine.

4. Serve the Mediterranean falafel bowl and savor the flavors!

Prep Time: 20 minutes

These hearty grain bowls offer a combination of textures, flavors, and nutrients that make for a satisfying lunch. You can customize these bowls by adding your favorite proteins, vegetables, or dressings to suit your preferences. Enjoy the wholesome goodness of these grain bowls and fuel your day with nourishing ingredients!

- Satisfying Wraps and Sandwiches

Let's look into filling wraps and sandwiches that are ideal for a quick and delectable lunch. These portable dinners are practical, adaptable, and flavorful. You may choose from a wide range of alternatives to satiate your cravings, whether you want a wrap or a traditional sandwich. Let's look at some enticing dishes to make your lunchtime more enjoyable!

Ingredients:
- One substantial whole wheat tortilla or wrap
 - 4-6 ounces of sliced, cooked chicken breast
 - 1/4 cup cucumbers, diced
   - 2 pieces of crumbled feta cheese - 1/4 cup of chopped tomatoes - 2 teaspoons of plain Greek yogurt
 - 1 teaspoon dried oregano - 1 tablespoon lemon juice
 - Add salt and pepper to taste - Sliced olives and fresh parsley are optional extras

- Requirements:
 1. To make the sauce, mix together the Greek yogurt, lemon juice, dried oregano, salt, and pepper in a small dish.

 2. Place the wrap or tortilla made from whole wheat on a flat surface.

 3. Evenly cover the tortilla or wrap with the Greek yogurt sauce.

 4. On top of the sauce, arrange the sliced chicken breast, chopped cucumbers, diced tomatoes, crumbled feta cheese, and any other ingredients.

 5. Tuck the wrap's edges in as you carefully roll it up.

 6. If preferred, cut the wrap in half diagonally and fasten with toothpicks.

Ten minutes for preparation

The Caprese Sandwich

Ingredients:
-two pieces of whole grain bread, a big tomato cut, and a few slices of fresh mozzarella cheese
1 tablespoon of balsamic glaze and fresh basil leaves
Extra virgin olive oil, 1 tablespoon
- To taste, salt and pepper

- **Requirements:**
1. Spread olive oil and balsamic glaze on one piece of bread.
2. Arrange the tomato slices, fresh basil leaves, and slices of mozzarella cheese on top.
3. Season to taste with salt and pepper.
4. Add the last piece of bread on top.
5. If preferred, cut the sandwich in half.
6. Five minutes to prepare

Veggie Wrap with Hummus

Ingredients
- One substantial whole wheat tortilla or wrap
1/2 cup of shredded carrots and 2-3 tablespoons of hummus
- 1/2 cup sliced (any color) bell peppers
- 1/4 cup of cucumber slices
- A little amount of mixed greens or baby spinach
- To taste, salt and pepper

- Requirements:

1. Place the wrap or tortilla made from whole wheat on a flat surface.

2. Cover the tortilla or wrap with the hummus in an equal layer.

3. Arrange the baby spinach or mixed greens, bell pepper slices, cucumber slices, and carrot shreds on top.

4. Season to taste with salt and pepper.

5. Tuck the wrap's edges in as you carefully roll it up.

6. If preferred, cut the wrap in half diagonally and fasten with toothpicks.

Ten minutes for preparation

These filling sandwiches and wraps have a delicious medley of tastes and textures, making them ideal for a filling meal.

Add your preferred spreads, veggies, or meats to the components to suit your tastes. Enjoy these delicious treats on the go as a filling and practical dinner choice!

- Flavorsome Soups and Stews

When the weather becomes chilly or you're in the mood for a big supper, these warming and nutritious meals are ideal. You'll discover a range of dishes to please your palate, from traditional favorites to exotic surprises. In this article, we'll look at five enticing soup and stew dishes that will make you feel warm and satiated.

Traditional chicken noodle soup

Ingredients:
  - 1 tablespoon olive oil - 1 diced onion - 2 sliced carrots
  - 2 cut celery stalks
  2 cups of cooked, shredded chicken and 4 cups of chicken broth
  - One cup of egg noodles.
  1 tsp. dried thyme
  - Season with salt and pepper to taste - Garnish with fresh parsley

- **Requirements**:
  1. In a big saucepan set over medium heat, warm the olive oil. Include the chopped celery, carrots, and onion. Cook the veggies until they are tender.
  2. Add the chicken broth and heat through.
  3. Include the egg noodles, dried thyme, shredded chicken, salt, and pepper. Noodles should be cooked until soft.
  4. Before serving, garnish with fresh parsley.
  5. 15 minutes to prepare.
  6. 30 minutes for cooking

Spicy Black Bean Soup

Ingredients:
 -2 tablespoons of olive oil, 1 chopped onion, 2 minced garlic cloves, and 2 washed and drained cans of black beans.
 -1 tomato dice from a can
 - 1/2 teaspoon chili powder - 1 teaspoon cumin - 1 cup vegetable broth
 - 1/4 teaspoon cayenne pepper (for more spice, if desired)
 Fresh cilantro for garnish, salt, and pepper to taste. Lime wedges for serving.

- **Requirements**:
 1. In a big saucepan set over medium heat, warm the olive oil. Add the minced garlic and onion, both chopped. Cook until tender and aromatic.
 2. Include the cumin, chili powder, cayenne pepper (if using), salt, and pepper along with the black beans, chopped tomatoes, vegetable broth. To blend, stir.
 3. After the soup comes to a boil, turn down the heat and simmer it for approximately 20 minutes to let the flavors blend.
 4. Garnish with lime juice and fresh cilantro before serving hot.
 5. Ten minutes to prepare
 6. 30 minutes for cooking

Creamy Basil Tomato Soup

Ingredients:
-2 tablespoons butter, 1 diced onion, 2 minced garlic cloves.
-2 chopped tomatoes in cans
- 1/2 cup heavy cream - 1 cup vegetable broth
- Tomato paste, 2 teaspoons
- 1/4 cup finely chopped fresh basil leaves
- To taste-tested salt and pepper - Garnished with croutons

- **Requirements:**
1. In a big saucepan over medium heat, melt the butter. Add the minced garlic and onion, both chopped. Cook onions until they are aromatic and transparent.

2. Include the tomato paste, heavy cream, tomato broth, chopped tomatoes, salt, and pepper. Stir well.

3. Bring the mixture to a boil before turning the heat down and allowing it to simmer for 15 to 20 minutes.

4. Combine the freshly cut basil leaves.

5. Blend the soup until it is smooth and creamy using an immersion blender or by transferring it to a blender.

6. When serving, top with more fresh basil leaves and croutons, if preferred.

7. Ten minutes for preparation

8. 30 minutes for cooking

Moroccan lentil stew

Ingredients:
2 tablespoons of extra virgin olive oil, 1 chopped onion, 2 sliced carrots, 2 sliced celery stalks, and 2 minced garlic cloves.

 1 teaspoon tomato paste

 - 1 teaspoon each of ground cumin and ground coriander

 - 1/4 teaspoon cinnamon - 1/2 teaspoon ground turmeric

 - 1 cup red lentils, dry

 4 cups vegetable broth, salt, and pepper to taste. Garnish with fresh cilantro.

- Requirements:

1. In a big saucepan set over medium heat, warm the olive oil. Include the minced garlic, sliced carrots, sliced celery, and chopped onion. Cook the veggies until they are tender.

2. Add the tomato paste along with the ground cinnamon, cumin, coriander, and turmeric. Cook until aromatic for one minute.

3. Include the veggie broth and dry red lentils. Bring to a boil, then lower the heat and simmer for 20 to 25 minutes, or until the lentils are cooked through.

4. To taste, add salt and pepper to the dish.

5. Garnish with fresh cilantro before serving hot.

6. 15 minutes to prepare.

7. 30 minutes for cooking

Mushroom soup with cream

Ingredients:
- 2 tablespoons butter - 1 chopped onion - 8 ounces sliced mushrooms
- 2 minced garlic cloves
- 1 cup heavy cream - 2 cups vegetable broth
- 1 teaspoon of all-purpose flour
1 tsp. dried thyme
- Season with salt and pepper to taste - Garnish with fresh parsley

- **Requirements**:
1. In a big saucepan over medium heat, melt the butter. Add the mushroom slices and the chopped onion. Cook until onions are tender and mushrooms are browned.

2. After cooking for a further minute, add the minced garlic.

3. Add salt, pepper, heavy cream, dried thyme, all-purpose flour, and vegetable broth. Stirring periodically, bring to a simmer, and cook for approximately 10 minutes.

4. Blend the soup until it is smooth and creamy using an immersion blender or by transferring it to a blender.

5. Garnish with fresh parsley before serving hot.

6. Ten minutes to prepare

7. 25 minutes for cooking

These delectable stews and soups will warm your heart and satiate your palate. Enjoy these healthful and delectable meals while indulging in the scents and soothing tastes.

Chapter 4: Snacks for Nursing Moms on the Go

- Homemade Energy Bars and Bites

Whether you need a quick pick-me-up between nursing sessions or a convenient snack to take with you on your daily activities, these homemade energy bars and bites are the perfect solution. Packed with wholesome ingredients and customizable to suit your taste preferences, these snacks will provide you with a boost of energy and nutrition. Let's explore a variety of recipes for delicious and nourishing homemade energy bars and bites!

1. Peanut Butter and Oat Energy Bars

- **Ingredients**:
  - 1 cup old-fashioned oats
  - 1/2 cup natural peanut butter
  - 1/4 cup honey or maple syrup
  - 1/4 cup chopped nuts (e.g., almonds, walnuts)
  - 1/4 cup dried fruits (e.g., raisins, cranberries)
  - 1/4 cup mini chocolate chips (optional)
  - 1 teaspoon vanilla extract
  - Pinch of salt

- Instructions:

1. In a mixing bowl, combine the oats, peanut butter, honey or maple syrup, chopped nuts, dried fruits, mini chocolate chips (if using), vanilla extract, and salt.

2. Stir well until all the ingredients are evenly incorporated.

3. Transfer the mixture to a lined baking dish and press it down firmly.

4. Refrigerate for at least 2 hours to allow the bars to set.

5. Once firm, cut into bars or bite-sized pieces.

6. Prep Time: 10 minutes

7. Refrigeration Time: 2 hours

2. Almond Date Energy Balls

- Ingredients:
- 1 cup pitted dates
- 1 cup raw almonds
- 2 tablespoons unsweetened cocoa powder
- 1 tablespoon chia seeds
- 1 tablespoon almond butter
- 1 teaspoon vanilla extract
- Pinch of salt
- Desiccated coconut or crushed almonds for rolling (optional)

- **Instructions**:
1. Place the dates, almonds, cocoa powder, chia seeds, almond butter, vanilla extract, and salt in a food processor.
2. Pulse until the ingredients are well combined and the mixture comes together into a sticky dough.
3. Scoop out small portions of the mixture and roll them into bite-sized balls.
4. If desired, roll the energy balls in desiccated coconut or crushed almonds for added texture and flavor.
5. Place the energy balls in an airtight container and refrigerate for at least 30 minutes to firm up.
6. Enjoy as a quick and nourishing snack on the go.
7. **Prep Time: 15 minutes**
8. **Refrigeration Time: 30 minutes**

3. No-Bake Cranberry Pistachio Bars

- **Ingredients:**
  - 1 cup pitted dates
  - 1 cup dried cranberries
  - 1 cup raw pistachios
  - 1/4 cup almond butter
  - 1/4 cup honey or maple syrup
  - 1 teaspoon vanilla extract
  - Pinch of salt

- **Instructions:**

1. In a food processor, combine the dates, dried cranberries, pistachios, almond butter, honey or maple syrup, vanilla extract, and salt.

2. Pulse until the ingredients are finely chopped and well combined.

3. Transfer the mixture to a lined baking

dish and press it down firmly.

4. Refrigerate for at least 1 hour to allow the bars to set.

5. Once chilled and firm, cut into bars or squares.

6. **Prep Time: 10 minutes**

7. **Refrigeration Time: 1 hour**

4. Apricot Coconut Energy Bites

- **Ingredients:**
  - 1 cup dried apricots
  - 1 cup unsweetened shredded coconut
  - 1/2 cup raw cashews
  - 2 tablespoons coconut oil, melted
  - 1 tablespoon honey or maple syrup
  - 1 teaspoon vanilla extract
  - Pinch of salt

- **Instructions:**

1. Place the dried apricots, shredded coconut, cashews, coconut oil, honey or maple syrup, vanilla extract, and salt in a food processor.

2. Pulse until the mixture is finely chopped and sticks together when pressed between your fingers.

3. Scoop out small portions of the mixture and roll them into bite-sized balls.

4. Place the energy bites on a baking sheet lined with parchment paper and refrigerate for 30 minutes to set.

5. Store in an airtight container in the refrigerator until ready to enjoy.

6. Prep Time: 15 minutes

7. Refrigeration Time: 30 minutes

5. Chocolate Chip Quinoa Bars

- Ingredients:
- 1 cup cooked quinoa
- 1/2 cup almond butter
- 1/4 cup honey or maple syrup
- 1/4 cup unsweetened shredded coconut
- 1/4 cup mini chocolate chips
- 1/4 cup chopped nuts (e.g., pecans, almonds)
- 1 teaspoon vanilla extract
- Pinch of salt

- Instructions:

1. In a mixing bowl, combine the cooked quinoa, almond butter, honey or maple syrup, shredded coconut,

mini chocolate chips, chopped nuts, vanilla extract, and salt.

2. Stir well until all the ingredients are evenly mixed.

3. Transfer the mixture to a lined baking dish and press it down firmly.

4. Refrigerate for at least 1 hour to allow the bars to set.

5. Once firm, cut into bars or squares.

6. Prep Time: 10 minutes

7. Refrigeration Time: 1 hour

These homemade energy bars and bites are not only delicious but also packed with essential nutrients to fuel your busy days as a nursing mom. They are a great option for a quick and nutritious snack whenever you need an energy boost. Feel free to experiment with different ingredients and flavors to suit your preferences. Enjoy the convenience and satisfaction of these homemade snacks on the go!

- Nut and Seed Trail Mixes

Let's look at a different great portable food for nursing mothers: nut and seed trail mixes. These mixtures are not only tasty and filling, but they are also rich in vital nutrients, giving you enduring energy all day. Nuts and seeds are an excellent option for a healthful snack since they include a broad variety of vitamins, minerals, healthy fats, and protein. Let's get started with these tasty and wholesome nut and seed trail mix recipes!

Traditional Nut Medley

Ingredients:
-1 cup cashews and 1 cup raw almonds.
 1-cup of walnuts
 One cup of pecans
 - A serving of dried cranberries
 - Half a cup of pumpkin seeds
 - A half-cup of sunflower seeds
 - One-fourth teaspoon sea salt

- Requirements:
  1. Combine the dried cranberries, almonds, cashews, walnuts, pecans, pumpkin seeds, sunflower seeds, and sea salt in a mixing dish.
  2. Gently stir the mixture until all the ingredients are spread equally.
  3. Put the trail mix In a storage container that is airtight.
  4. Take a few anytime you want a fast and wholesome snack.
  5. Five minutes to prepare

Tropical Paradise Blend

Ingredients:
 -1 cup unsweetened coconut flakes and 1 cup raw cashews.
 - 1 cup dried mango slices - 1 cup dried pineapple pieces
 - 1/2 cup banana chips - 1/2 cup macadamia nuts
 1-fourth cup of chia seeds

- **Requirements:**
 1. Combine the cashews, coconut flakes, pieces of dried pineapple, slices of dried mango, macadamia nuts, banana chips, and chia seeds in a mixing dish.
 2. Gently stir everything together until well-combined.
 3. Put the trail mix in a storage container that is airtight.
 4. Take this cocktail with you everywhere you go for a taste of heaven.
 5. Five minutes to prepare

Flavored Seed Mix

Ingredients:
 -1 cup raw almonds, 1 cup sunflower seeds, and 1 cup pumpkin seeds.
 - Half a cup of sesame seeds

- 1/4 cup maple syrup or honey
- 1 tablespoon melted coconut oil
- 1 teaspoon cinnamon, ground

  1/4 teaspoon of grated nutmeg and 1/2 teaspoon of ground ginger
- One-fourth teaspoon sea salt

- Requirements:

Almonds, pumpkin seeds, sunflower seeds, sesame seeds, honey or maple syrup, melted coconut oil, ground cinnamon, crushed ginger, ground nutmeg, and sea salt should all be combined in a mixing dish.

2. Stir the ingredients together until the seeds and nuts are well covered.

3. Evenly distribute the seed mixture on a baking sheet covered with parchment paper.

4. Bake for 15 to 20 minutes at 325 °F (165 °C), or until brown and aromatic.

5. Take it out of the oven, let it cool fully, and then put it in an airtight container.

6. Eat this savory and crispy spiced seed mixture as a snack or top yogurt or salads with it.

7. Ten minutes for preparation

8. Bake for 15 minutes.

Sweet-salty mixture

Ingredients:

1 cup each of raw cashews, almonds, and peanuts.
- One cup of broken-up pretzel sticks

- Half a cup of dried cranberries
- 1/2 cup chips of dark chocolate
- 2 teaspoons of maple syrup or honey
- 1/4 teaspoon sea salt - 1 teaspoon vanilla extract

- **Requirements:**
1. Combine the dark chocolate chips, pretzel sticks, dried cranberries, honey or maple syrup, vanilla essence, and sea salt in a mixing dish.
2. Continue tossing the mixture until the sweet and salty combination is uniformly distributed over all of the components.
3. Put the trail mix in a storage container that is airtight.
4. Snack on this delicious mixture of sweet and salty ingredients for a filling treat.
5. Five minutes to prepare

Superfood Mix of Seeds

Ingredients:
-1 cup each of hemp seeds, chia seeds, and flax seeds
- Half a cup of goji berries
- 1/2 cup blueberries, dried
Cacao nibs, 1/4 cup
- 1/4 cup coconut meat, shredded

- **Requirements:**

1. Combine the hemp seeds, chia seeds, flax seeds, dried blueberries, goji berries, cacao nibs, and shredded coconut in a mixing dish.

2. Combine well until each component is spread equally.

3. Put the trail mix in a storage container that is airtight.

4. This superfood seed mix is full of nutrients and may be eaten as a snack or added to porridge or smoothies.

5. Five minutes to prepare

In addition to being practical, these homemade nut and seed trail mixes provide a variety of tastes and textures to meet your snacking requirements. You are welcome to alter the mixtures to suit your tastes by adding or removing elements. Enjoy these nutrient-rich snacks while you're on the road to provide you the strength and sustenance you need to be a breastfeeding mother.

- Guilt-Free Sweet Treats

Being a nursing mother should not prevent you from indulging in delectable sweets. With these recipes, you can satisfy your sweet needs while still feeding your child and yourself healthier alternatives to typical treats. Let's investigate a selection of delicious and wholesome sweet treat recipes that are guilt-free!

1. Avocado with Chocolate Mousse

Ingredients

2 ripe avocados and 1/4 cup unsweetened chocolate powder are the ingredients.

- 1/4 cup honey or maple syrup
- One-fourth cup almond milk
– One teaspoon of vanilla extract
- A dash of salt
- Optional garnishes include berries, coconut shavings, and chopped almonds.

- Requirements:

1. Combine the avocados, cocoa powder, maple syrup or honey, almond milk, vanilla extract, and sea salt in a blender or food processor.

2. Add all ingredients to a blender and process until creamy and well-blended.

3. Place serving plates or glasses with the mousse inside.

4. Allow it set in the refrigerator for at least an hour.

5. Add your preferred garnish, such as fresh berries, coconut shavings, or chopped almonds.

6. Feel free to indulge in this luscious and rich chocolate avocado mousse!

7. Ten minutes for preparation

8. One hour of chilling time

2. Chia Berry Pudding

- ingredients

1-fourth cup of chia seeds

- 1 cup almond milk or any other kind of milk you want.

- 1 tablespoon maple syrup or honey

- Fresh berries for the topping - 1/2 teaspoon vanilla essence

- Requirements:

1. Combine the chia seeds, almond milk, maple syrup or honey, and vanilla essence in a bowl.

2. Be careful to thoroughly stir to incorporate the chia seeds into the liquid.

3. Stir the mixture once more to avoid clumping after letting it settle for approximately 5 minutes.

4. To enable the chia seeds to gel and take on the consistency of pudding, cover the bowl and place it in the refrigerator for at least two hours or overnight.

5. To guarantee a smooth texture and break up any clumps, give the pudding a vigorous stir just before serving.

6. Add fresh berries or other toppings of your choice.

7. Enjoy this berry chia pudding as a guilt-free dessert or snack. It is hydrating and nourishing.

8. Five minutes for preparation

9. Relaxation Period: Two Hours

3.Banana Oat Cookies

Ingredients:

2 mashed, ripe bananas

- 1 1/2 cups of rolled oats - 1/4 cup of your preferred nut butter, such as almond butter

- 2 teaspoons of maple syrup or honey

– One teaspoon of vanilla extract

- Option to add chips of bittersweet chocolate, chopped nuts, and dried fruit

- Requirements:

1. Set a baking sheet on your oven's 350°F (175°C) rack and preheat the oven.

2. Combine the mashed bananas with the rolled oats, almond butter, honey, maple syrup, and vanilla extract in a mixing dish.

3. Make sure to completely combine all the components by vigorously stirring.

4. If preferred, stir in your add-in of choice, such as chopped nuts, dark chocolate chips, or dried fruit.

distributed.

5. Drop rounded amounts of the dough onto the prepared baking sheet using a tablespoon or cookie scoop.

6. Using the back of a spoon or your fingers, gently press each part into the dish.

7. Bake the cookies for 12 to 15 minutes, or until the sides are lightly browned.

8. Take them out of the oven and let them cool for a little while on the baking sheet before transferring them to a wire rack to finish cooling.

9. Enjoy these healthy and filling banana oat biscuits as a treat.

10. Ten minutes for preparation

11. Bake for 12 to 15 minutes

4. Coconut Bliss Balls

Ingredients:

- 1/2 cup almond flour or crushed almonds - 1 cup unsweetened shredded coconut

- 1/4 cup melted coconut oil

- 2 teaspoons of maple syrup or honey

– One teaspoon of vanilla extract

- A dash of salt

- Extra coconut shavings, cocoa powder, and crushed nuts are optional coatings.

- Requirements:

1. Combine the ground or ground almonds, melted coconut oil, honey, maple syrup, vanilla essence, and sea salt in a mixing dish.

2. Combine all the ingredients by properly combining them.

3. Scoop out little amounts of the mixture and form them into balls that are suitable for a bite.

4. To add more flavor and texture, roll the balls, as desired, in more shredded coconut, cocoa powder, or ground almonds.

5. To set the bliss balls, place them on a baking sheet covered with parchment paper and put the sheet in the fridge for 30 minutes.

6. Prior to serving, store in the refrigerator in an airtight container.

7. Enjoy these coconut happiness balls as a tasty treat without feeling bad.

8. 15 minutes for preparation

9. 30-minute refrigeration period

5. Apples with Cinnamon Baked

Ingredients:

- 4 apples, cored (we recommend Granny Smith or Honeycrisp).

- 2 tablespoons melted butter or coconut oil

- 2 teaspoons of maple syrup or honey

- 1 teaspoon cinnamon, ground

Greek yogurt, raisins, and chopped almonds are available as extras.

- Requirements:

1. Set the oven's temperature to 375°F (190°C).

2. Combine the melted coconut oil or butter, honey or maple syrup, and ground cinnamon in a small bowl.

3. Arrange the cored apples on a prepared baking sheet or baking dish.

4. Evenly cover the apples with the cinnamon mixture by drizzling it over them.

5. If desired, load the apple cores with your preferred garnishes, such as raisins or chopped almonds.

6. Bake the apples for 20 to 25 minutes, or until they are soft and have started to caramelize.

7. Take them out of the oven, and then give them some time to cool.

8. You can serve the baked apples alone or with some Greek yogurt on top for extra richness.

9. Savor the soothing tastes and natural sweetness of these baked apples guilt-free.

10. Ten minutes for preparation

11. Bake for 20 to 25 minutes

As a nursing mother, these guilt-free sweet snacks provide you healthful options to sate your sweet appetite while maintaining a healthy and balanced diet. With the knowledge that you are giving yourself and your child healthy and delectable indulgence alternatives, you may enjoy these tasty meals guilt-free.

- Savory Grab-and-Go Snacks

savory grab-and-go snacks ideal for nursing mothers who are busy. These snacks not only taste good and fill you up, but they also provide you a nutrition and energy boost to get you through the rest of the day. These savory snacks are guaranteed to satisfy your cravings, whether you're looking for a fast snack in between meals or a handy alternative for traveling. Let's explore some tasty choices!

1. Mini Quiches with Veggies

Ingredients include:
- four eggs.
1/4 cup of milk
- 1/2 cup chopped veggies, such as spinach, bell peppers, and mushrooms
- 1/4 cup grated cheese, preferably feta or cheddar
- To taste, salt and pepper

- Requirements:
1. Lightly oil a tiny muffin tray and preheat your oven to 375°F (190°C).
2. Combine the milk and eggs in a mixing dish by thoroughly whisking them together.
3. Add the shredded cheese, diced veggies, salt, and pepper.
4. Fill each cavity in the tiny muffin tray that has been prepared approximately 3/4 full with the mixture.
5. Bake the quiches for 15 to 18 minutes, or until they are set and have a light golden brown top.
6. Let them cool a little before taking them out of the muffin tray.

7. These small quiches with packed vegetables are the ideal fast and tasty snack.

8. Ten minutes to prepare

9. Bake for 15 to 18 minutes

2. Pinwheels of spinach and feta

- ingredients

- 1 sheet of thawed puff pastry

- 1/4 cup feta cheese that has been crumbled; - 1 cup of fresh spinach leaves; - 1/4 teaspoon of garlic powder

- To taste, salt and pepper

- Requirements:

1. Set your oven to 400 degrees Fahrenheit (200 degrees Celsius) and cover a baking sheet with parchment paper.

2. Shape the puff pastry into a rectangle on a lightly dusted surface.

3. Evenly distribute the fresh spinach leaves on the puff pastry.

4. Top the spinach with the feta cheese crumbles, garlic powder, salt, and pepper.

5. Form the puff pastry into a log by carefully rolling it up from one end.

6. Cut the log into pinwheels that are 1/2 inch thick using a sharp knife.

7. Arrange the pinwheels on the lined baking sheet, leaving space between each one.

8. Bake the pinwheels for 15 to 18 minutes, or until they are puffy and brown.

9. Before serving, allow them to cool somewhat.

10. These pinwheels of spinach and feta make a tasty and handy snack.

11. 15 minutes for preparation

12. Bake for 15 to 18 minutes.

3. Wraps with Mediterranean hummus

Ingredients:
- 4 tortillas made with whole wheat
- 1 cup of mixed greens or lettuce - 1 cup of hummus
- 1/2 cup cucumbers, diced
- 1/2 cup tomatoes, diced
- One-fourth cup of sliced Kalamata olives
- 2 tablespoons feta cheese, crumbled
- To taste, salt and pepper

Instructions

1. Spread out the whole-wheat tortillas on a spotless surface.

2. Cover each tortilla with a thick layer of hummus and spread it out equally.

3. Add chopped Kalamata olives, diced tomatoes, diced cucumbers, mixed greens or lettuce, and crumbled feta cheese on top.

4. To taste, add salt and pepper to the dish.

5. Tightly roll the tortillas, folding the edges in as you go.

6. If preferred, divide each wrap in half or make bite-sized chunks.

7. These hummus wraps from the Mediterranean region are the ideal fast and filling snack.

8. Ten minutes to prepare

4. Small Caprese Skewers

Ingredients:
Cherry or grape tomatoes, fresh mozzarella balls, fresh basil, and optional balsamic drizzle.

- Requirements:
1. To assemble the small caprese skewers, thread a cherry or grape tomato, a ball of fresh mozzarella, and a leaf of fresh basil onto a skewer.

2. Continue until you have as many skewers as you need.

3. To provide a taste boost, drizzle with balsamic glaze, if preferred.

4. These little caprese skewers make for an easy and light snack.

5. Five minutes to prepare

5. Cinnamon-Roasted Chickpeas

Ingredients:
1 can washed and drained chickpeas; 1 tablespoon extra-virgin olive oil; 1 teaspoon chile powder.

- A half teaspoon of paprika

- Half a teaspoon of garlic powder
cayenne pepper, 1/4 teaspoon (adjust to taste)
- A pinch of salt

- **Requirements**:

1. Set your oven to 400 degrees Fahrenheit (200 degrees Celsius) and cover a baking sheet with parchment paper.

2. To eliminate extra moisture, pat the chickpeas dry with a paper towel.

3. Combine the chickpeas with salt, olive oil, cayenne pepper, paprika, chili powder, and garlic powder in a bowl.

4. Evenly distribute the seasoned chickpeas on the lined baking sheet.

5. Bake the chickpeas for 20 to 25 minutes, stirring once, or until they are crispy and golden brown.

6. Let these hot roasted chickpeas cool before consuming.

7. Five minutes to prepare

8. Bake for 20 to 25 minutes.

You have a variety of alternatives with these tasty grab-and-go snacks to fill your day with scrumptious and healthful bits. These recipes have you covered whether you're seeking for protein-rich dishes, sweets filled with vegetables, or travel-friendly wraps. As you manage the requirements of nursing and the hectic life of a mom on the move, take pleasure in the ease of these flavorful snacks.

Chapter 5: Nourishing Dinners for Mom and Family

- Wholesome One-Pot Meals

Healthful one-pot dishes are designed to energize mom and the whole family. These dinners are not only quick and easy, but they also include a lot of healthy components that will encourage breastfeeding and provide everyone at the table a well-balanced meal. Let's delve into the warm and tasty realm of satisfying one-pot dinners!

1. Stir-fried chicken and vegetables

Ingredients:
1 tablespoon chopped ginger, 2 cloves of minced garlic, 2 teaspoons sesame oil, 2 boneless, skinless chicken breasts, sliced bell peppers, sliced, in a cup
- broccoli florets, 1 cup
- 1/4 cup low-sodium soy sauce or tamari - 2 tablespoons honey or maple syrup - 1 cup snap peas
   - Sesame seeds and sliced green onions are extra garnishes.

- **Requirements:**

1. In a big skillet or wok, heat the sesame oil over medium-high heat.

2. Add the chicken breast slices, and heat them through and until browned. Take out of the skillet, then put it aside.

3. Add the minced ginger and garlic to the same pan and cook for a minute, or until fragrant.

4. Include the broccoli florets, snap peas, and bell pepper slices in the pan. Vegetables should be stir-fried for 3–4 minutes to achieve tender-crispness.

5. Combine the honey or maple syrup and low-sodium soy sauce (or tamari) in a small bowl.

6. After adding the sauce to the pan of veggies, toss them together.

7. Return the cooked chicken to the pan and stir to evenly distribute the sauce.

8. Continue cooking for one more minute, or until the chicken is fully heated.

9. Arrange the chicken and vegetable stir-fry on top of quinoa or steamed rice.

10. To add flavor and garnish, top with sliced green onions and sesame seeds.

11. Delight in this filling one-pot dinner that combines protein, vegetables, and savory spices.

12. 15 minutes for preparation

13. 15 minutes for cooking

2. Curry with lentils and vegetables

Ingredients:
1 tablespoon coconut oil, 1 chopped onion, 2 minced garlic cloves.
- 2 teaspoons curry powder - 1 tablespoon grated ginger
- 1 cup washed red lentils
-1 coconut milk can
2 cups of chopped vegetables, such as carrots, bell peppers, and zucchini, and 2 cups of vegetable broth
Optional garnishes include fresh cilantro and a squeeze of lime juice.

- Requirements:
1. Place a big saucepan over medium heat and warm the coconut oil.
2. Include the grated ginger, minced garlic, and chopped onion in the saucepan. The onion should be transparent and aromatic after sautéing.
3. Add the curry powder and stir. Toast the spices for one more minute.
4. Fill the saucepan with the lentils that have been washed, coconut milk, vegetable broth, and chopped veggies. To blend, thoroughly stir.
5. Once the mixture has reached a boil, turn the heat down to low and cover the pan.
6. Simmer the lentils and veggies for 20 to 25 minutes, or until they are soft.
7. To taste, add salt and pepper to the dish.

8. Over cooked rice or quinoa, serve the lentil and vegetable curry.

9. For a blast of freshness, garnish with fresh cilantro and a squeeze of lime juice.

10. Treat your family to this hearty, nutrient-dense one-pot supper.

11. 10 minutes for preparation

12. 25 minutes for cooking

3. Skillet with quinoa and black beans

Ingredients:

- 1 tablespoon olive oil - 1 diced onion - 1 diced bell pepper - 2 minced garlic cloves

- 1 cup washed quinoa

- 2 cups of vegetable broth - 1 can of washed and drained black beans

- 1/2 teaspoon paprika - 1 teaspoon cumin

Salt and pepper to taste; possible toppings include avocado slices and fresh cilantro minced. 1/4 teaspoon chile powder

- Requirements:

1. In a big pan over medium heat, warm the olive oil.

2. Add the minced garlic, onion, and bell pepper to the skillet. Sauté the veggies until they are tender.

3. Add the vegetable broth, black beans, cumin, paprika, and chili powder (if using) after the quinoa has been rinsed. Mix thoroughly.

4. Once the mixture has reached a rolling boil, turn the heat down to low and cover the skillet.

5. Let the quinoa simmer for 15 to 20 minutes, or until it is cooked and the liquid has been absorbed.

6. To taste, add salt and pepper.

7. Alternatively, you may top the quinoa and black bean pan with avocado slices and fresh cilantro that has been chopped.

8. Delight in this filling and healthy one-pot dish that is bursting with plant-based protein.

9. Ten minutes to prepare

10. 20 minutes for cooking

4. Foil packets with salmon and vegetables

Ingredients:
2 salmon filets, 2 cups mixed veggies (including cherry tomatoes, bell peppers, and asparagus),

- 1 tablespoon lemon juice - 2 teaspoons olive oil

- 1 teaspoon dried dill - Salt and pepper to taste - Fresh parsley as an optional garnish

- **Requirements**:
1. Set the oven's temperature to 400°F (200°C).

Each salmon filet should be placed on a sizable piece of aluminum foil.

3. Set the salmon filets in the center of the mixed veggies.

4. Drizzle the fish and veggies with the olive oil and lemon juice.

5. Season with salt and pepper and add dried dill.

6. To make a package, fold the foil over the salmon and veggies and seal the edges.

7. Place the foil packages on a baking sheet and bake for 15 to 20 minutes, or until the salmon is fully cooked and the veggies are soft.

8. Open the foil packages with caution, being mindful of the steam.

9. If preferred, garnish with fresh parsley.

10. As a wonderful and healthy supper alternative, serve these foil packs of salmon and vegetables.

11. 10 minutes for preparation

12. Bake for 15 to 20 minutes.

5. Coconut curry with vegetables and chickpeas

- ingredients

Coconut oil, 1 tbsp

- 1 chopped onion - 2 minced garlic cloves

- 2 teaspoons curry powder - 1 tablespoon grated ginger

- 1 can coconut cream

2 cups of vegetable broth, 2 cups of diced vegetables (such as sweet potatoes, cauliflower, and carrots), 1 can of rinsed and drained chickpeas, salt, and pepper to taste are optional additions.

- **Requirements:**

1. Place a big saucepan over medium heat and warm the coconut oil.

2. Include the grated ginger, minced garlic, and chopped onion in the saucepan. The onion should be transparent and aromatic after sautéing.

3. Add the curry powder and stir. Toast the spices for one more minute.

4. Add the chickpeas, coconut milk, vegetable broth, and diced veggies to the saucepan. To blend, thoroughly stir.

5. Once the mixture has reached a boil, turn the heat down to low and cover the pan.

6. Simmer the veggies for 20 to 25 minutes, or until they are soft.

7. To taste, add salt and pepper to the dish.

8. Spoon the cooked rice or quinoa over the coconut curry with chickpeas and vegetables.

9. To add more flavor, garnish with chopped fresh cilantro and a squeeze of lime juice.

10. Delight in this delectable and wholesome one-pot dish that combines the virtues of veggies and chickpeas in a creamy coconut curry sauce.

11. 10 minutes for preparation

12. 25 minutes for cooking

Mom and the whole family are nourished and satisfied by these healthy one-pot dinners. These dinners are ideal for busy nursing women who want to provide healthful and balanced meals to their loved ones because of their delectable tastes, nutrient-rich ingredients, and simple preparation. Take advantage of the simplicity and nutrition of these one-pot miracles while you enjoy nursing and family mealtimes.

-Flavorful Sheet Pan Dinners

Let us look at the collection of flavorful sheet pan dinners that make mealtime a breeze. These recipes are designed to provide nourishing and balanced meals for both breastfeeding moms and the whole family, all cooked on a single sheet pan for easy cleanup. Let's dive into the world of delicious and hassle-free sheet pan dinners!

1. Lemon Herb Roasted Chicken with Vegetables

- **Ingredients**:
  - 4 bone-in, skin-on chicken thighs
  - 2 tablespoons olive oil
  - 1 tablespoon lemon juice
  - 2 cloves garlic, minced
  - 1 teaspoon dried thyme
  - 1 teaspoon dried rosemary
  - Salt and pepper to taste

- 2 cups mixed vegetables (such as potatoes, carrots, Brussels sprouts)

- **Instructions:**
1. Preheat your oven to 400°F (200°C) and line a sheet pan with parchment paper.

2. In a small bowl, combine the olive oil, lemon juice, minced garlic, dried thyme, dried rosemary, salt, and pepper.

3. Place the chicken thighs on the prepared sheet pan and brush the herb mixture evenly over each piece.

4. Toss the mixed vegetables in any remaining herb mixture, then arrange them around the chicken on the sheet pan.

5. Roast in the preheated oven for 30-35 minutes or until the chicken is cooked through and the vegetables are tender.

6. Serve the lemon herb roasted chicken with vegetables as a satisfying and flavorful sheet pan dinner.

7. Prep Time: 10 minutes

8. Cooking Time: 30-35 minutes

2. Teriyaki Salmon and Broccoli

- **Ingredients:**
  - 2 salmon filets
  - 2 cups broccoli florets
  - 1/4 cup teriyaki sauce
  - 2 tablespoons honey or maple syrup

- 1 tablespoon soy sauce or tamari
- 1 tablespoon sesame oil
- 1 teaspoon grated ginger
- 1 clove garlic, minced
- Optional toppings: sesame seeds, sliced green onions

- **Instructions:**
1. Preheat your oven to 400°F (200°C) and line a sheet pan with parchment paper.
2. Place the salmon filets in the center of the prepared sheet pan.
3. Arrange the broccoli florets around the salmon.
4. In a small bowl, whisk together the teriyaki sauce, honey or maple syrup, soy sauce or tamari, sesame oil, grated ginger, and minced garlic.
5. Pour the teriyaki sauce mixture over the salmon and broccoli, coating them evenly.
6. Bake in the preheated oven for 12-15 minutes or until the salmon is cooked to your desired doneness and the broccoli is tender-crisp.
7. Sprinkle with sesame seeds and sliced green onions, if desired.
8. Serve the teriyaki salmon and broccoli as a delicious and nutritious sheet pan dinner option.
9. **Prep Time: 10 minutes**
10. **Cooking Time: 12-15 minutes**

3. Mediterranean Veggie Bake

- **Ingredients:**
  - 2 cups cherry tomatoes
  - 1 zucchini, sliced
  - 1 yellow bell pepper, sliced
  - 1 red onion, sliced
  - 2 tablespoons olive oil
  - 2 cloves garlic, minced
  - 1 teaspoon dried oregano
  - 1 teaspoon dried basil
  - Salt and pepper to taste
  - 1/2 cup crumbled feta cheese
  - Optional garnish: fresh basil leaves

- **Instructions:**
  1. Preheat your oven to 400°F (200°C) and line a sheet pan with parchment paper.
  2. Place the cherry tomatoes, zucchini slices, yellow bell pepper slices, and red onion slices on the prepared sheet pan.
  3. Drizzle with olive oil and sprinkle minced garlic, dried oregano, dried basil, salt, and pepper over the vegetables. Toss to coat evenly.
  4. Roast in the preheated oven for 20-25 minutes or until the vegetables are tender.

5. Sprinkle the crumbled feta cheese over the roasted vegetables and return to the oven for an additional 2-3 minutes to slightly melt the cheese.

6. Garnish with fresh basil leaves, if desired.

7. Serve the Mediterranean veggie bake as a vibrant and flavorful sheet pan dinner.

8. Prep Time: 10 minutes

9. Cooking Time: 20-25 minutes

4. Spiced Shrimp and Vegetable Fajitas

- **Ingredients:**
  - 1 pound shrimp, peeled and deveined
  - 1 red bell pepper, sliced
  - 1 green bell pepper, sliced
  - 1 yellow onion, sliced
  - 2 tablespoons olive oil
  - 1 tablespoon chili powder
  - 1 teaspoon ground cumin
  - 1/2 teaspoon smoked paprika
  - Salt and pepper to taste
  - Tortillas and desired toppings (such as avocado, salsa, sour cream)

- **Instructions:**
  1. Preheat your oven to 400°F (200°C) and line a sheet pan with parchment paper.
  2. In a small bowl, combine the chili powder, ground cumin, smoked paprika, salt, and pepper.

3. Place the shrimp, bell pepper slices, and onion slices on the prepared sheet pan.

4. Drizzle with olive oil and sprinkle the spice mixture over the shrimp and vegetables. Toss to coat evenly.

5. Roast in the preheated oven for 8-10 minutes or until the shrimp are pink and cooked through, and the vegetables are tender-crisp.

6. Warm the tortillas according to package instructions.

7. Serve the spiced shrimp and vegetable fajitas on the warmed tortillas with desired toppings.

8. Enjoy these flavorful and satisfying fajitas as a delicious sheet pan dinner.

9. Prep Time: 10 minutes

10. Cooking Time: 8-10 minutes

5. Herb-Roasted Tofu and Vegetables

- Ingredients:

- 1 block tofu, pressed and cut into cubes

- 2 cups mixed vegetables (such as broccoli, cauliflower, carrots)

- 2 tablespoons olive oil

- 1 tablespoon soy sauce or tamari

- 1 teaspoon dried thyme

- 1 teaspoon dried rosemary

- Salt and pepper to taste

- Instructions:

1. Preheat your oven to 400°F (200°C) and line a sheet pan with parchment paper.

2. Place the tofu cubes and mixed vegetables on the prepared sheet pan.

3. Drizzle with olive oil and soy sauce or tamari. Sprinkle dried thyme, dried rosemary, salt, and pepper over the tofu and vegetables. Toss to coat evenly.

4

. Roast in the preheated oven for 25-30 minutes or until the tofu is golden and the vegetables are tender.

5. Serve the herb-roasted tofu and vegetables as a wholesome and plant-based sheet pan dinner.

6. Prep Time: 10 minutes

7. Cooking Time: 25-30 minutes

These flavorful sheet pan dinners in Chapter 5 offer a variety of options to nourish and satisfy both mom and the whole family. With minimal preparation and easy cleanup, these meals are perfect for busy breastfeeding moms who want to enjoy wholesome and delicious dinners without spending too much time in the kitchen. Embrace the convenience and deliciousness of these sheet pan dinners as you continue your breastfeeding journey and create memorable family meals.

- Protein-Rich Entrees

Let's explore a variety of protein-packed dishes that provide vital nutrition to families and nursing mothers. These dishes provide a range of alternatives to accommodate various dietary demands and tastes while still being tasty and fulfilling. Let's investigate these filling and energizing dishes that are high in protein!

Lemon-Herb Grilled Chicken Breast

Ingredients

Four boneless, skinless chicken breasts make up the ingredients.
- 2 tablespoons of olive oil - 1 lemon's juice
- 2 minced garlic cloves
- 1 teaspoon each of dried thyme and rosemary
- To taste, salt and pepper

- Requirements:
1. Turn the grill's heat up to medium-high.
2. Mix the olive oil, lemon juice, minced garlic, dried thyme, dried rosemary, salt, and pepper in a small bowl.
3. Pour the marinade over the chicken breasts in a shallow dish, being sure to coat them completely. Wait at least 30 minutes before serving.

4. Grill the chicken breasts for 6 to 8 minutes on each side, or until they register 165°F (75°C) inside.

5. Take the food off the grill and set it aside to rest before serving.

6. To complete a protein-rich supper, slice the grilled lemon-herb chicken breasts and serve them with your preferred sides or salads.

7. 10 minutes for preparation + marinating time

8. Preparation Time: 12 to 16 minutes

2. Salmon baked in a lemon-dill sauce

Ingredients:

1 lemon juice, 2 tablespoons olive oil, 4 fish filets
  two tablespoons of dried dill, salt, and pepper to taste

- Requirements:

1. Line a baking sheet with parchment paper and preheat the oven to 400°F (200°C).

On the prepared baking sheet, arrange the salmon filets.

3. Combine the olive oil, lemon juice, dried dill, salt, and pepper in a small bowl.

4. Cover the salmon filets with the lemon-dill sauce, being sure to cover them completely.

5. Bake the salmon in the preheated oven for 12 to 15 minutes, depending on how done you want it.

6. For a wholesome and protein-rich meal, serve the baked salmon with the lemon-dill sauce with steamed vegetables or a side salad.

7. Ten minutes for preparation

8. Preparation Time: 12 to 15 minutes

3. Bell Peppers Stuffed with Quinoa and Black Beans

Ingredients

- 4 bell peppers of any hue.

- 1 cup black beans that have been cooked; - 1 cup quinoa; - 1 cup chopped tomatoes

- 1/2 cup corn kernels - 1/2 cup sliced red onion

- Half a cup of crumbled cheddar cheese (or a dairy-free substitute)

- 1 teaspoon each of ground cumin and paprika

- To taste, salt and pepper

- Requirements:

1. Grease a baking dish and preheat the oven to 375°F (190°C).

2. Cut the bell peppers' tops off, then scoop out the seeds and membranes.

3. Mix everything in a large mixing dish, the black beans, chopped tomatoes, red onion, corn, shredded cheddar cheese, quinoa that has been cooked, as well as salt, pepper, cumin, and paprika. Blend well.

4. Gently push down the quinoa and black bean filling into the bell peppers.

5. Place the foil-shrouded filled bell peppers in the oiled baking tray.

6. Bake for 30-35 minutes in a preheated oven, or until the mixture is well cooked and the bell peppers are soft.

7. Take off the foil, cover with more shredded cheddar cheese (if wanted), and bake for a further 5 minutes, or until the cheese is bubbling and melted.

8. As a filling and protein-rich supper meal, serve the quinoa and black bean filled bell peppers.

9. 20 minutes for preparation

10. Preparation Time: 35 to 40 minutes

4. Stir-Fried Tofu with Vegetables

Ingredients:

2 tablespoons soy sauce or tamari, 1 tablespoon hoisin sauce, 1 block diced and pressed tofu.

- 1 tablespoon each of rice vinegar, sesame oil, and cornstarch. - 2 tablespoons each of vegetable oil.

- 2 chopped garlic cloves - 1 inch piece of grated ginger - 1 sliced bell pepper

Snap peas and broccoli florets in equal portions, with salt and pepper to taste

- Requirements:

In order to make a marinade, combine the soy sauce or tamari, hoisin sauce, rice vinegar, sesame oil, and cornstarch in a basin.

2. Combine the marinade with the tofu cubes, mix to coat, and let alone for 10 to 15 minutes.

3. In a large skillet or wok, heat the vegetable oil over medium-high heat.

4. To the pan, add the minced garlic and the grated ginger, and cook for one to two minutes, or until fragrant.

5. Add the marinated tofu to the pan and cook for 5-7 minutes, or until golden brown on both sides, while saving the marinade.

6. Take the tofu out of the pan and put it aside.

7. Include the bell pepper, broccoli florets, snap peas, and any other chosen veggies in the same skillet. Vegetables should be stir-fried for 3–4 minutes to achieve tender-crispness.

8. Add the tofu back to the pan with the veggies, and then cover with the marinade that was set aside. Stir-fry for a further 2 to 3 minutes, or until everything is well cooked and coated.

9. To taste, add salt and pepper to the dish.

10. As a tasty and protein-rich entrée, serve the tofu stir-fry with veggies. If preferred, serve it with steamed rice or noodles.

11. 20 minutes for preparation

12. Preparation Time: 15 to 20 minutes

5. Curry with lentils and vegetables

Ingredients:

1 cup rinsed and drained dry lentils; 1 chopped onion; 2 minced garlic; 1 grated ginger; and 1 chopped bell pepper.

- 1 diced carrot
- 1 diced zucchini
- One 14-ounce can of coconut milk
Curry powder, 2 teaspoons
- 1 teaspoon each of ground cumin and turmeric
- To taste, salt and pepper
- Optional garnish of fresh cilantro

- Requirements:

1. Heat a tablespoon of oil in a big saucepan over medium heat.

2. Include the chopped onion and heat until transparent and tender.

3. Stir in the grated ginger and minced garlic, and cook for one more minute.

4. Add the bell pepper, carrot, and zucchini that have been cut, and sauté for a few minutes until they start to soften.

5. Fill the saucepan with the coconut milk, curry powder, cumin and turmeric powders, salt, and pepper.

6. Bring the ingredients to a boil, then lower the heat to a simmer, cover the pan, and cook the lentils for 20 to 25 minutes, depending on how soft you want your lentils.

7. Taste and, if necessary, adjust the seasoning.

8. Top the lentil and vegetable curry with fresh cilantro, if preferred, and serve with naan bread or over steaming rice.

9. 15 minutes to prepare.

10. 30 minutes for cooking

These recipes provide a tasty and balanced method to fulfill your nutritional requirements while taking pleasure in nourishing meals with your family, whether you choose chicken, fish, plant-based proteins, or legumes. Explore the alternatives available and find new favorites as you go with nursing.

- Plant-Powered Delights

Let us celebrate the incredible flavors and nourishment that plant-based ingredients can provide. These plant-powered delights are not only packed with essential nutrients, but they also offer a wonderful array of colors, textures, and flavors that will delight your taste buds. Whether you're a dedicated vegan or simply looking to incorporate more plant-based meals into your diet, these recipes will inspire and satisfy. Let's dive into the world of plant-powered delights!

1. Roasted Vegetable Buddha Bowl

- **Ingredients:**
  - 1 cup cooked quinoa
  - Assorted vegetables (such as sweet potatoes, broccoli, cauliflower, carrots, bell peppers), chopped
  - 2 tablespoons olive oil
  - 1 teaspoon smoked paprika
  - 1/2 teaspoon cumin
  - Salt and pepper to taste
  - Mixed greens or spinach
  - Avocado slices
  - Tahini dressing (optional)

- **Instructions:**
  1. Preheat the oven to 425°F (220°C) and line a baking sheet with parchment paper.
  2. In a large bowl, toss the chopped vegetables with olive oil, smoked paprika, cumin, salt, and pepper until well-coated.
  3. Spread the vegetables in a single layer on the prepared baking sheet.
  4. Roast in the preheated oven for 20-25 minutes, or until the vegetables are tender and slightly caramelized.

5. While the vegetables are roasting, assemble your Buddha bowl by layering cooked quinoa, mixed greens or spinach, roasted vegetables, and avocado slices.

6. Drizzle with tahini dressing if desired.

7. Enjoy this nourishing and vibrant plant-powered delight!

2. Lentil and Spinach Curry

- **Ingredients:**
  - 1 cup dried red lentils, rinsed and drained
  - 1 onion, chopped
  - 2 cloves garlic, minced
  - 1-inch piece ginger, grated
  - 1 tablespoon curry powder
  - 1 teaspoon ground cumin
  - 1 teaspoon ground coriander
  - 1 can (14 ounces) diced tomatoes
  - 1 can (14 ounces) coconut milk
  - 2 cups fresh spinach leaves
  - Salt and pepper to taste
  - Fresh cilantro for garnish (optional)

- **Instructions:**
  1. In a large pot, heat a tablespoon of oil over medium heat.

  2. Add the chopped onion and cook until softened and translucent.

3. Add the minced garlic, grated ginger, curry powder, ground cumin, and ground coriander, and sauté for another minute until fragrant.

4. Stir in the rinsed lentils, diced tomatoes, and coconut milk.

5. Bring the mixture to a boil, then reduce the heat to low, cover the pot, and let simmer for 15-20 minutes, or until the lentils are tender and cooked through.

6. Stir in the fresh spinach leaves and cook for an additional 2-3 minutes until wilted.

7. Season with salt and pepper to taste.

8. Garnish with fresh cilantro if desired.

9. Serve the lentil and spinach curry with steamed rice or naan bread for a satisfying and flavorful plant-powered meal.

3. Portobello Mushroom Burgers

- Ingredients:
- 4 large portobello mushroom caps
- 4 whole grain burger buns
- 1/4 cup balsamic vinegar
- 2 tablespoons olive oil
- 2 cloves garlic, minced
- 1 teaspoon dried thyme
- Salt and pepper to taste
- Toppings of your choice (lettuce, tomato, onion, avocado, etc.)

- Instructions:

1. In a small bowl, whisk together the balsamic vinegar, olive oil, minced garlic, dried thyme, salt, and pepper to create a marinade.

2. Place the portobello mushroom caps in a shallow dish and pour the marinade over them. Let them marinate for at least 15 minutes, flipping them halfway through.

3. Preheat a grill or grill pan over medium-high heat.

4. Grill the marinated portobello mushroom caps for about 4-5 minutes on each side, or until they are tender and lightly charred.

5. Toast the burger buns on the grill for a minute or two, until lightly toasted.

6. Assemble your portobello mushroom burgers by placing each grilled mushroom cap on a burger bun and adding your desired toppings.

7. Serve these plant-powered delights with a side of sweet potato fries or a fresh salad for a satisfying and wholesome dinner.

4. Chickpea and Vegetable Stir-Fry

- Ingredients:
- 1 can (15 ounces) chickpeas, rinsed and drained
- 1 red bell pepper, sliced
- 1 yellow bell pepper, sliced
- 1 zucchini, sliced
- 1 carrot, sliced

- 1 cup snap peas
- 2 cloves garlic, minced
- 1-inch piece ginger, grated
- 3 tablespoons soy sauce or tamari
- 2 tablespoons hoisin sauce
- 1 tablespoon sesame oil
- 1 tablespoon cornstarch
- Cooked rice or noodles for serving

- **Instructions:**

1. In a small bowl, whisk together the soy sauce or tamari, hoisin sauce, sesame oil, and cornstarch to create a sauce.

2. Heat a tablespoon of oil in a large skillet or wok over medium-high heat.

3. Add the minced garlic and grated ginger to the skillet and sauté for 1-2 minutes until fragrant.

4. Add the sliced bell peppers, zucchini, carrot, snap peas, and chickpeas to the skillet and stir-fry for 3-4 minutes until the vegetables are tender-crisp.

5. Pour the sauce over the stir-fried vegetables and chickpeas, stirring well to coat everything evenly.

6. Continue cooking for another 2-3 minutes until the sauce thickens slightly.

7. Serve the chickpea and vegetable stir-fry over cooked rice or noodles for a quick and nutritious plant-powered dinner.

Chapter 6: Boosting Milk Supply with Lactation-Friendly Recipes

- Lactation Smoothies and Shakes

Let us delve into the delightful world of lactation-friendly dishes to help nursing mothers increase their milk production. We are aware that nursing mothers place a high importance on keeping a plentiful milk supply, and that proper nutrition is essential to attaining this objective. These shakes and smoothies for breastfeeding are not only tasty but also loaded with nutrients that promote lactation. Let's look at some nutritional dishes that might support you when you are nursing.

Bliss Lactation Smoothie

Ingredients:
- 1 ripe banana - 1 cup mixed berries (strawberries, blueberries, and raspberries)
- 1 tsp. flaxseed meal
Brewer's yeast, 1 tablespoon
- 1 cup kale or spinach
– 1 cup almond milk (or other kind of milk)

- Optional additional sweetness: 1-2 tablespoons of honey or maple syrup

- **Requirements:**
1. Blend the spinach or kale, almond milk, flaxseed meal, brewer's yeast, mixed berries, ripe banana, and sweetener (if using) in a blender.
2. Blend at maximum speed until creamy and smooth.
3. Pour the smoothie into a glass and enjoy the revitalizing and lactation-enhancing effects.

Lactation Shake with Peanut Butter and Banana

Ingredients:
-1 banana that is ripe.
- 2 teaspoons of peanut butter - 1 teaspoon of chia seeds
- 1 tablespoon brewer's yeast - 1 cup of your preferred milk (dairy or vegan).
– 1-2 tablespoons maple syrup or honey (optional)
- Ice cubes, if desired

- **Requirements:**
1. Blend the ripe banana with the peanut butter, chia seeds, brewer's yeast, milk, sweetener, and ice cubes (if using) in a blender.
2. Blend until creamy and smooth.

3. Pour into a glass and enjoy this lactation-enhancing shake's nutty and filling tastes.

Green Power Lactation Smoothie

Ingredients:
-1 cup of fresh spinach, 1 pear that has been cored and diced, and 1/2 an avocado.
- 1 tsp. flaxseed meal
Brewer's yeast, 1 tablespoon
- 1 cup water or coconut water
Juice from half a lemon
– 1-2 tablespoons maple syrup or honey (optional)

- Requirements:
1. Blend the coconut water or water, fresh spinach, ripe pear, avocado, flaxseed meal, brewer's yeast, lemon juice, and sweetener (if using) in a blender.
2. Blend until creamy and smooth.
3. Pour the green power smoothie into a glass and enjoy its energizing and lactation-enhancing qualities.

Lactation Chocolate Banana Shake

Ingredients:
-1 banana that is ripe.
- 2 tablespoons chocolate powder, unsweetened

- 1 teaspoon of almond butter
Brewer's yeast, 1 tablespoon
- 1 cup of your preferred milk (dairy or vegan).
– 1-2 tablespoons maple syrup or honey (optional)
- Ice cubes, if desired

- Requirements:
1. Blend the ripe banana with the milk, brewer's yeast, cocoa powder, almond butter, sweetener of choice, and ice cubes (if using) in a blender.
2. Blend until creamy and smooth.
3.Pour yourself a glass and savor the decadent chocolate tastes of this smoothie that helps in lactation.

Tropical Delight Milk Smoothie

Ingredients:
-1 ripe banana, 1/2 cup sliced pineapple, and 1/2 cup sliced mango.
- 1 tablespoon flaxseed meal, 1 tablespoon coconut oil
Brewer's yeast, 1 tablespoon
- 1 cup water or coconut water
– 1-2 tablespoons maple syrup or honey (optional)

- Requirements:
1. Blend the coconut oil, flaxseed meal, brewer's yeast, ripe banana, pineapple pieces, mango chunks, coconut water or water, and sweetener (if preferred) in a blender.
2. Blend until creamy and smooth.

3. Pour this revitalizing and lactation-enhancing smoothie into a glass, and escape to a tropical paradise.

These lactation shakes and smoothies provide important nutrients to maintain a healthy milk production in addition to being a delightful treat. Always pay attention to your body's signals and change the ingredients as necessary to fit your taste preferences and nutritional needs. Enjoy these delectable dishes and feed your body while feeding your child.

- Galactagogue-Infused Snacks

These galactagogue-infused snacks are specifically designed to support lactation and boost milk supply for breastfeeding moms. Galactagogues are substances that promote milk production, and incorporating them into snacks can be a convenient and delicious way to enhance your breastfeeding journey. Let's take a closer look at these nutritious and lactation-boosting snack ideas.

1. Oatmeal Lactation Cookies

Oatmeal is a well-known galactagogue that is rich in iron, fiber, and antioxidants. These oatmeal lactation cookies not only provide a tasty treat but also help promote healthy milk production. They often include ingredients like brewer's yeast, flaxseed meal, and fenugreek, which are additional galactagogues known to support lactation.

2. Date and Almond Lactation Energy Balls

Dates and almonds are both considered galactagogues and are packed with essential nutrients. These energy balls offer a convenient and nutritious snack option for busy breastfeeding moms. They are often made by blending dates, almonds, oats, and other ingredients such as coconut oil, honey, or nut butter. These bite-sized snacks provide a quick energy boost and can help support milk supply.

3. Lactation Granola Bars

Granola bars infused with galactagogues can be a convenient on-the-go snack for nursing moms. They often contain a combination of oats, nuts, seeds, and galactagogue-rich ingredients like brewer's yeast, flaxseed, or fenugreek. These bars provide a satisfying and nourishing snack option while supporting lactation.

4. Chia Seed Pudding

Chia seeds are known for their high omega-3 fatty acid content and are often included in lactation-friendly snacks. Chia seed pudding is a popular choice as it is easy to prepare and can be customized with various flavors and toppings. Combine chia seeds, milk of your choice, sweetener, and galactagogue ingredients like brewer's yeast or fenugreek for a creamy and nutritious snack.

5. Nut Butter and Galactagogue-Infused Toast

A simple yet satisfying snack option is spreading your favorite nut butter on toast and adding galactagogue-infused toppings. Nut butters like almond butter or peanut butter provide healthy fats and protein, while adding galactagogue ingredients like sliced bananas, flaxseeds, or sesame seeds can further enhance the lactation-boosting properties of this snack.

These galactagogue-infused snacks not only offer a variety of flavors and textures but also provide important nutrients to support breastfeeding and milk production. Remember to consult with a healthcare professional or lactation consultant to ensure the ingredients are suitable for your individual needs and any potential allergies or sensitivities. Enjoy these delicious and nourishing snacks as part of your breastfeeding journey.

- Milk-Boosting Main Courses

Milk-Boosting Main Courses

The collection of milk-boosting main courses are specially designed to support lactation and provide nourishment for breastfeeding moms. These recipes feature ingredients known as galactagogues, which promote milk production and ensure a healthy milk supply. Let's explore these delicious and nutritious milk-boosting main course ideas.

1. Salmon with Dill and Lemon

Salmon is not only a great source of lean protein but also contains omega-3 fatty acids, which are beneficial for both mom and baby. This recipe combines fresh salmon filets with the flavors of dill and lemon for a light and refreshing main course. Serve it alongside a side of steamed vegetables or a whole grain pilaf for a well-rounded and milk-boosting meal.

2. Spinach and Chickpea Curry

Leafy green vegetables like spinach are known to be rich in calcium, iron, and other essential nutrients for breastfeeding moms. This flavorful spinach and chickpea curry combines the goodness of spinach with protein-packed chickpeas and a blend of aromatic spices. Serve it over brown rice or with whole wheat naan bread for a satisfying and milk-boosting dinner.

3. Quinoa and Vegetable Stir-Fry

Quinoa is a nutritious grain that provides a complete protein source and is high in fiber. This quinoa and vegetable stir-fry recipe incorporates colorful and nutrient-rich vegetables, such as bell peppers, broccoli, and carrots, for a balanced and wholesome main course. Seasoned with soy sauce or tamari and garnished with toasted sesame seeds, this dish offers a delicious and milk-boosting option for breastfeeding moms.

4. Lentil and Vegetable Soup

Lentils are an excellent source of plant-based protein, iron, and fiber, making them an ideal ingredient for milk-boosting main courses. This lentil and vegetable soup combines lentils with a variety of vegetables, such as carrots, celery, and tomatoes, for a hearty and nourishing meal. Serve it with a side of whole grain bread for a complete and satisfying dinner.

5. Chicken and Sweet Potato Curry

Chicken is a lean protein source that provides essential amino acids for milk production. This chicken and sweet potato curry recipe pairs tender chicken pieces with creamy sweet potatoes and a fragrant blend of spices. The combination of protein and complex carbohydrates in this dish makes it a milk-boosting main course option for breastfeeding moms.

These milk-boosting main courses not only provide essential nutrients for lactation but also offer a variety of flavors and textures to keep mealtime exciting. Remember to adjust the recipes to suit your dietary preferences and consult with a healthcare professional or lactation consultant if you have any specific concerns or dietary restrictions. Enjoy these nourishing meals as you continue your breastfeeding journey.

- Sweet Indulgences for Milk Production

The selection of sweet indulgences is not only to satisfy your cravings but also support milk production for breastfeeding moms. These recipes are crafted with ingredients known as galactagogues, which can help enhance lactation and ensure a healthy milk supply. Let's explore these delightful sweet treats that can nourish both your taste buds and your breastfeeding journey.

1. Oatmeal Chocolate Chip Lactation Cookies

Oatmeal is a well-known galactagogue that provides essential nutrients like iron and fiber. These delicious lactation cookies combine the wholesome goodness of oats with the sweetness of chocolate chips. Additionally, they often include ingredients like brewer's yeast and flaxseed, which further support milk production. Enjoy a warm, freshly baked cookie as a sweet and lactation-boosting treat.

2. Banana Bread with Galactagogue Twist

Banana bread is a beloved classic, and when infused with galactagogue ingredients, it becomes a nutritious and milk-boosting dessert. This recipe combines ripe bananas with ingredients like brewer's yeast, fenugreek, or flaxseed meal to enhance its lactation benefits. Enjoy a slice of this moist and flavorful bread as a guilt-free indulgence.

3. Berry Chia Seed Pudding

Chia seeds are a nutritional powerhouse, packed with omega-3 fatty acids and fiber. When combined with sweet and tangy berries, they create a delectable chia seed pudding. This creamy and dairy-free dessert is not only a refreshing treat but also provides essential nutrients to support lactation. Prepare it in advance and enjoy it as a healthy and indulgent snack or dessert option.

4. Dark Chocolate Energy Bites

Dark chocolate contains antioxidants and minerals like iron and magnesium, making it a delightful and beneficial addition to lactation-friendly sweets. These energy bites are made with dates, nuts, and a generous amount of dark chocolate, providing a satisfying and nutritious treat. Enjoy a couple of these bite-sized delights to satisfy your sweet tooth and boost milk production.

5. Coconut Milk Rice Pudding

Coconut milk is a rich source of healthy fats and can provide a creamy base for a lactation-boosting rice pudding. This recipe combines cooked rice, coconut milk, sweetener of choice, and aromatic spices like cinnamon and cardamom. The result is a comforting and flavorful dessert that not only satisfies your sweet cravings but also supports milk production.

These sweet indulgences offer a range of flavors and textures while incorporating galactagogue ingredients to enhance lactation. Remember to enjoy them in moderation as part of a balanced diet and consult with a healthcare professional or lactation consultant for any specific concerns or dietary considerations. Treat yourself to these delightful sweets while nourishing your breastfeeding journey.

Chapter 7: Quick and Easy Meals for Busy Moms

- 15-Minute Meals

In Chapter 7 of our cookbook, we focus on providing quick and easy meal solutions for busy moms. We understand that time is precious, especially for mothers juggling multiple responsibilities. These 15-minute meals are designed to be efficient, yet still nutritious and delicious. Let's explore these time-saving recipes that will help you whip up satisfying meals in no time.

1. Lemon Garlic Shrimp Stir-Fry

- **Ingredients:**
  - 1 pound shrimp, peeled and deveined
  - 2 tablespoons olive oil
  - 4 cloves garlic, minced
  - 1 teaspoon lemon zest
  - 2 tablespoons lemon juice
  - 1 cup mixed vegetables (such as bell peppers, broccoli, and snap peas)
  - Salt and pepper to taste
  - Optional: soy sauce or teriyaki sauce for extra flavor

- **Instructions:**

1. In a large skillet or wok, heat the olive oil over medium-high heat.

2. Add the minced garlic and sauté for about 1 minute until fragrant.

3. Add the shrimp to the skillet and cook for 2-3 minutes on each side until pink and cooked through.

4. Stir in the lemon zest, lemon juice, and mixed vegetables. Cook for an additional 2-3 minutes until the vegetables are tender-crisp.

5. Season with salt and pepper to taste. If desired, drizzle with soy sauce or teriyaki sauce for added flavor.

6. Serve the stir-fry over steamed rice or noodles for a quick and satisfying meal.

2. Caprese Salad with Grilled Chicken

- Ingredients:
  - 2 boneless, skinless chicken breasts
  - 2 tablespoons balsamic vinegar
  - 2 tablespoons olive oil
  - Salt and pepper to taste
  - 2 cups cherry tomatoes, halved
  - 8 ounces fresh mozzarella cheese, sliced
  - Fresh basil leaves, torn
  - Optional: balsamic glaze for drizzling

- Instructions:
  1. Preheat a grill or grill pan over medium-high heat.

2. Season the chicken breasts with balsamic vinegar, olive oil, salt, and pepper.

3. Grill the chicken for about 6-8 minutes per side until cooked through.

4. Remove the chicken from the grill and let it rest for a few minutes. Slice it into thin strips.

5. In a large bowl, combine the cherry tomatoes, fresh mozzarella slices, and torn basil leaves.

6. Arrange the sliced chicken over the tomato and mozzarella mixture.

7. Drizzle with balsamic glaze if desired.

8. Serve the Caprese salad with grilled chicken as a light and refreshing meal.

3. Turkey and Veggie Wrap

- Ingredients:
- 4 large whole wheat tortillas
- 8 ounces sliced turkey breast
- 1 cup mixed salad greens
- 1/2 cup sliced cucumber
- 1/2 cup sliced bell peppers
- 1/4 cup hummus or your favorite spread

- Instructions:
1. Lay out the tortillas and spread a tablespoon of hummus or spread of your choice onto each tortilla.

2. Layer the sliced turkey, mixed salad greens, cucumber slices, and bell pepper slices evenly on each tortilla.

3. Tightly roll up the tortillas, folding in the sides as you go.

4. Slice the wraps in half and secure with toothpicks if needed.

5 Serve the turkey and veggie wraps as a quick and portable meal.

4. Quinoa and Black Bean Salad

- **Ingredients**:
  - 2 cups cooked quinoa
  - 1 can black beans, drained and rinsed
  - 1 cup diced tomatoes
  - 1 cup diced cucumbers
  - 1/2 cup diced red onion
  - 1/4 cup chopped fresh cilantro
  - Juice of 1 lime
  - 2 tablespoons olive oil
  - Salt and pepper to taste

- **Instructions**:
  1. In a large bowl, combine the cooked quinoa, black beans, diced tomatoes, diced cucumbers, diced red onion, and chopped fresh cilantro.

  2. In a small bowl, whisk together the lime juice, olive oil, salt, and pepper.

3. Drizzle the dressing over the quinoa and black bean mixture and toss to combine.

4. Adjust the seasoning if needed.

5. Serve the quinoa and black bean salad as a nutritious and satisfying meal.

5. Veggie Egg Scramble

- Ingredients:
- 4 large eggs
- 1/2 cup diced bell peppers
- 1/2 cup diced tomatoes
- 1/4 cup diced onion
- 1/4 cup chopped spinach
- Salt and pepper to taste
- Optional toppings: shredded cheese, sliced avocado, salsa

- Instructions:
1. In a medium bowl, whisk the eggs until well beaten.

2. Heat a non-stick skillet over medium heat.

3. Add the diced bell peppers, tomatoes, and onion to the skillet and sauté for 2-3 minutes until slightly softened.

4. Add the chopped spinach to the skillet and cook for an additional 1-2 minutes until wilted.

5. Pour the beaten eggs over the vegetable mixture in the skillet.

6. Gently scramble the eggs with a spatula until they are cooked to your desired consistency.

7. Season with salt and pepper to taste.

8. Serve the veggie egg scramble with optional toppings like shredded cheese, sliced avocado, or salsa.

These 15-minute meals are designed to save you time while still providing nourishing and satisfying options for busy moms. Feel free to customize the recipes with your preferred ingredients or adapt them to suit your dietary preferences. Enjoy these quick and easy meals as a delicious solution for those hectic days.

- Instant Pot Delights

The Instant Pot is a versatile kitchen appliance that can help busy moms create delicious and flavorful meals in a fraction of the time compared to traditional cooking methods. These Instant Pot recipes are designed to save you time without compromising on taste. Let's explore the wonderful world of Instant Pot delights.

1. Tender and Juicy Pulled Chicken

- Ingredients:

- 2 pounds boneless, skinless chicken breasts or thighs

- 1 cup chicken broth
- 1/2 cup barbecue sauce
- 2 tablespoons apple cider vinegar
- 2 tablespoons honey
- 1 teaspoon smoked paprika
- 1/2 teaspoon garlic powder
- 1/2 teaspoon onion powder
- Salt and pepper to taste

- Instructions:

1. Place the chicken breasts or thighs in the Instant Pot.

2. In a bowl, whisk together the chicken broth, barbecue sauce, apple cider vinegar, honey, smoked paprika, garlic powder, onion powder, salt, and pepper.

3. Pour the sauce mixture over the chicken in the Instant Pot.

4. Close the lid and set the Instant Pot to the "Pressure Cook" or "Poultry" setting for 15 minutes.

5. Once the cooking time is complete, allow the pressure to release naturally for 5 minutes, then manually release any remaining pressure.

6. Use two forks to shred the chicken directly in the Instant Pot.

7. Serve the tender and juicy pulled chicken on buns, over rice, or as a filling for tacos or wraps.

2. Flavorful Lentil Soup

- Ingredients:
  - 1 cup dried lentils, rinsed and drained
  - 1 onion, chopped
  - 2 carrots, chopped
  - 2 celery stalks, chopped
  - 3 cloves garlic, minced
  - 1 can diced tomatoes
  - 4 cups vegetable broth
  - 1 teaspoon ground cumin
  - 1/2 teaspoon ground turmeric
  - 1/2 teaspoon smoked paprika
  - Salt and pepper to taste
  - Fresh cilantro or parsley for garnish (optional)

- Instructions:
1. Place the lentils, chopped onion, chopped carrots, chopped celery, minced garlic, diced tomatoes (with their juices), vegetable broth, ground cumin, ground turmeric, smoked paprika, salt, and pepper in the Instant Pot.
2. Stir well to combine.
3. Close the lid and set the Instant Pot to the "Soup" or "Manual" setting for 15 minutes.
4. Once the cooking time is complete, allow the pressure to release naturally for 10 minutes, then manually release any remaining pressure.

5. Give the lentil soup a good stir before serving.

6. Garnish with fresh cilantro or parsley if desired.

7. Serve the flavorful lentil soup hot with crusty bread or a side salad for a satisfying meal.

3. Creamy Tomato Basil Pasta

- Ingredients:
   - 8 ounces pasta (such as penne or rotini)
   - 1 can diced tomatoes
   - 1 onion, diced
   - 3 cloves garlic, minced
   - 2 cups vegetable broth
   - 1/2 cup heavy cream or coconut cream for a dairy-free option
   - 1/4 cup grated Parmesan cheese or nutritional yeast for a vegan option
   - 1/4 cup fresh basil leaves, chopped
   - Salt and pepper to taste

- Instructions:
   1. Place the pasta, diced tomatoes (with their juices), diced onion, minced garlic, and vegetable broth in the Instant Pot.

   2. Stir well to combine.

   3. Close the lid and set the Instant Pot to the "Manual" or "Pressure Cook" setting for half of the pasta's recommended cooking time (e.g., if the pasta usually takes 10 minutes, set the Instant Pot for 5 minutes).

4. Once the cooking time is complete, quick-release the pressure.

5. Stir in the heavy cream or coconut cream and grated Parmesan cheese or nutritional yeast.

6. Season with salt and pepper to taste.

7. Stir in the fresh chopped basil leaves.

8. Allow the sauce to thicken slightly before serving.

9. Serve the creamy tomato basil pasta hot with an extra sprinkle of Parmesan cheese or nutritional yeast.

4. Fluffy Quinoa Pilaf

- **Ingredients:**
  - 1 cup quinoa, rinsed and drained
  - 1 1/2 cups vegetable broth
  - 1 tablespoon olive oil
  - 1 onion, diced
  - 2 cloves garlic, minced
  - 1 bell pepper, diced
  - 1 zucchini, diced
  - 1 teaspoon ground cumin
  - 1/2 teaspoon ground turmeric
  - Salt and pepper to taste
  - Fresh parsley for garnish (optional)

- **Instructions:**
  1. Turn on the "Sauté" function on the Instant Pot and heat the olive oil.

2. Add the diced onion, minced garlic, diced bell pepper, and diced zucchini to the Instant Pot.

3. Sauté for a few minutes until the vegetables are slightly softened.

4. Add the rinsed quinoa, vegetable broth, ground cumin, ground turmeric, salt, and pepper to the Instant Pot.

5. Stir well to combine.

6. Close the lid and set the Instant Pot to the "Manual" or "Pressure Cook" setting for 1 minute.

7. Once the cooking time is complete, quick-release the pressure.

8. Fluff the quinoa pilaf with a fork.

9. Garnish with fresh parsley if desired.

10. Serve the fluffy quinoa pilaf as a delicious and nutritious side dish.

5. Tender Pot Roast

- Ingredients:
- 2 pounds beef chuck roast
- 2 tablespoons olive oil
- 1 onion, sliced
- 3 cloves garlic, minced
- 2 carrots, chopped
- 2 celery stalks, chopped
- 1 cup beef broth
- 1 tablespoon Worcestershire sauce
- 1 teaspoon dried thyme

- 1 teaspoon dried rosemary
- Salt and pepper to taste

- **Instructions:**
1. Season the beef chuck roast with salt and pepper.
2. Turn on the "Sauté" function on the Instant Pot and heat the olive oil.
3. Brown the roast on all sides in the Instant Pot.
4. Remove the roast from the Instant Pot and set it aside.
5. Add the sliced onion, minced garlic, chopped carrots, and chopped celery to the Instant Pot.
6. Sauté for a few minutes until the vegetables are slightly softened.
7. Return the roast to the Instant Pot, placing it on top of the vegetables.
8. Pour the beef broth and Worcestershire sauce over the roast

9. Sprinkle the dried thyme and dried rosemary over the roast.
10. Close the lid and set the Instant Pot to the "Manual" or "Pressure Cook" setting for 60 minutes.
11. Once the cooking time is complete, allow the pressure to release naturally for 10 minutes, then manually release any remaining pressure.
12. Remove the roast from the Instant Pot and let it rest for a few minutes before slicing.
13. Serve the tender pot roast with the cooked vegetables and drizzle with the flavorful juices.

These Instant Pot delights offer a wide variety of flavors and options to help you create quick and delicious meals for yourself and your family. Enjoy the convenience and efficiency of Instant Pot cooking while still enjoying wholesome and nourishing dishes.

- Freezer-Friendly Recipes

These recipes are designed to be prepared ahead of time and stored in the freezer, making them convenient options for busy moms. Whether you're looking to stock up on ready-to-eat meals or make-ahead ingredients, these freezer-friendly recipes have got you covered. Let's dive into the wonderful world of freezer-friendly cooking.

Freezer-Friendly Breakfast Burritos

- **Ingredients:**
  - 8 large flour tortillas
  - 8 large eggs
  - 1/2 cup diced bell peppers
  - 1/2 cup diced onions
  - 1/2 cup shredded cheese
  - Salt and pepper to taste
  - Optional add-ins: cooked bacon, sausage, or vegetables

- **Instructions:**
  1. In a bowl, whisk the eggs until well beaten.
  2. Heat a non-stick skillet over medium heat and scramble the eggs.
  3. Add the diced bell peppers, diced onions, shredded cheese, salt, and pepper to the scrambled eggs.
  4. Optional: Add cooked bacon, sausage, or vegetables as desired.
  5. Allow the filling to cool slightly.
  6. Spoon the egg filling onto each flour tortilla and roll them up tightly, folding in the sides to create a burrito shape.
  7. Wrap each breakfast burrito tightly in plastic wrap or aluminum foil.
  8. Place the wrapped burritos in a freezer-safe bag or container.
  9. Label the bag or container with the date and contents.
  10. Freeze the breakfast burritos for up to 3 months.
  11. When ready to eat, remove the desired number of burritos from the freezer and microwave for 2-3 minutes or until heated through.
  12. Enjoy a delicious and convenient breakfast on the go.

Freezer-Friendly Chicken and Vegetable Stir-Fry

- **Ingredients:**
  - 2 boneless, skinless chicken breasts, sliced
  - 2 cups mixed vegetables (such as bell peppers, broccoli, carrots, and snap peas)
  - 1/4 cup soy sauce
  - 2 tablespoons oyster sauce
  - 2 tablespoons hoisin sauce
  - 1 tablespoon sesame oil
  - 2 cloves garlic, minced
  - 1 teaspoon grated ginger
  - Salt and pepper to taste

- **Instructions:**
  1. Heat a large skillet or wok over medium-high heat.
  2. Add the sliced chicken breasts and cook until no longer pink.
  3. Add the mixed vegetables to the skillet and stir-fry for a few minutes until slightly tender.
  4. In a bowl, whisk together the soy sauce, oyster sauce, hoisin sauce, sesame oil, minced garlic, grated ginger, salt, and pepper.
  5. Pour the sauce over the chicken and vegetables in the skillet.

6. Stir-fry for another minute to coat everything evenly in the sauce.

7. Remove the skillet from the heat and allow the stir-fry to cool completely.

8. Divide the stir-fry into individual portions and transfer them to freezer-safe containers or bags.

9. Label the containers or bags with the date and contents.

10. Freeze the chicken and vegetable stir-fry for up to 3 months.

11. When ready to eat, thaw the desired portion in the refrigerator overnight.

12. Reheat in a skillet or microwave until heated through.

13. Serve over rice or noodles for a quick and flavorful meal.

Freezer-Friendly Spinach and Feta Stuffed Chicken Breasts

- **Ingredients:**
  - 4 boneless, skinless chicken breasts
  - 1 cup frozen spinach, thawed and squeezed dry
  - 1/2 cup crumbled feta cheese
  - 2 cloves garlic, minced
  - 1 tablespoon olive oil
  - Salt and pepper to taste

- **Instructions:**
   1. Preheat the oven to 375°F (190°C).
   2. In a bowl, combine the thawed spinach, crumbled feta cheese, minced garlic, olive oil, salt, and pepper.
   3. Cut a horizontal slit into each chicken breast to create a pocket.
   4. Stuff each chicken breast with the spinach and feta mixture.
   5. Season the outside of the chicken breasts with additional salt and pepper if desired.
   6. Place the stuffed chicken breasts on a baking sheet lined with parchment paper.
   7. Bake in the preheated oven for 25-30 minutes or until the chicken is cooked through and the filling is hot and bubbly.
   8. Allow the stuffed chicken breasts to cool completely.
   9. Individually wrap each chicken breast tightly in plastic wrap or aluminum foil.
   10. Place the wrapped chicken breasts in a freezer-safe bag or container.
   11. Label the bag or container with the date and contents.
   12. Freeze the spinach and feta stuffed chicken breasts for up to 3 months.
   13. When ready to eat, thaw the desired chicken breast in the refrigerator overnight.
   14. Reheat in the oven or microwave until heated through.
   15. Serve with a side of your choice for a satisfying and hassle-free dinner.

By preparing freezer-friendly recipes, you can save time and effort in the kitchen while still enjoying delicious and nutritious meals. These recipes are designed to be made ahead of time, frozen, and then easily reheated whenever you need them. From breakfast burritos to stir-fries and stuffed chicken breasts, these freezer-friendly options will keep you well-fed and satisfied even on your busiest days.

- Simple Meal Prep Ideas

Meal prepping is a great way to save time, lower stress, and make sure you have delicious and healthful meals available all week. This chapter offers you a range of food preparation suggestions that are simple to carry out and provide pleasing outcomes. Let's explore the realm of easy meal preparation and see how it may change the way you prepare.

1. Getting Ready Protein Options:

Making protein selections ahead of time is a crucial component of meal planning. This comprises marinating, preparing, and storing meats in portioned containers, such as chicken breasts, beef, or fish. To have protein sources throughout the week, you may also make a batch of hard-boiled eggs or cook a big pot of beans or lentils. You'll have the building blocks for healthy meals and save time throughout the week while preparing individual meals if you prepare protein alternatives.

2. Preparing and Chopping Veggies:

Vegetable preparation in advance, including chopping and dicing, is a crucial component of meal planning. Vegetables including bell peppers, carrots, cucumbers, and celery should be washed, peeled, and chopped before being stored in airtight containers or bags. You'll have prepared veggies on hand when it's time to cook in this manner, saving you valuable time during dinner preparation. These prepared vegetables may be added to salads, stir-fries, roasted vegetable meals, or eaten as snacks all week long.

3. Making Salads with Grains and Pasta:

Salads made of grains and pasta are adaptable and filling alternatives that can be made ahead of time and eaten all week long. Cook some grains, such as quinoa, brown rice, or couscous, then combine them with a choice of herbs, veggies, and dressing. To make fast dinners or simple grab-and-go lunches, store the salad in portioned containers. For a balanced dinner, you may add proteins like grilled chicken, tofu, or chickpeas to your grain and pasta salads.

4. Building salads in Mason jars:

Making salads in mason jars is an easy and aesthetically pleasing method to prepare your meals in advance. In a mason jar, layer salad greens, diced veggies, protein (such tofu or grilled chicken), nuts or seeds, and dressing. Shake the container to disperse the dressing when it's time to eat, then tuck into a crisp salad. The layering method preserves the freshness of the ingredients and stops them from becoming mushy.

5. Snack and trail mix portioning:

Not only do you prepare your major meals; you also prepare your snacks. When hunger hits, it's simple to grab a nutritious snack by portioning up foods like cut-up fruits, yogurt cups, almonds, or homemade trail mixes into individual containers or bags. This keeps you from mindlessly munching on less healthy foods and makes sure you always have healthful alternatives accessible.

You'll save time, lower your stress level, and maintain a nutritious diet by adopting these simple meal preparation ideas into your daily routine. Meal planning gives you the ability to remain organized and make thoughtful food decisions throughout the week whether you're preparing protein alternatives, slicing veggies, creating grain salads, putting together salads in mason jars, or portioning out snacks. Accept the idea of quick meal preparation and profit from quick, wholesome cooking.

Chapter 8: Desserts and Treats to Savor

- Guilt-Free Indulgences

It's crucial to occasionally reward yourself while leading a healthy lifestyle without sacrificing your dietary objectives. This chapter provides a variety of delectable sweets and snacks that are tasty, filling, and produced with healthy ingredients. Let's investigate the realm of guilt-free delights and learn how to enjoy delectable treats guilt-free.

Delicious Dark Chocolate Avocado Mousse

Ingredients
- two ripe avocados.
- 1/4 cup chocolate powder, unsweetened
- 1/4 cup pure honey or maple syrup
– One teaspoon of vanilla extract
– A dash of salt

Fresh berries, chopped almonds, or coconut shreds are available as extra toppings.

- Requirements:
1. Scoop the avocado flesh into a food processor or blender.
2. Include the salt, maple syrup, honey, vanilla essence, and chocolate powder.
3. Blend, scraping down the sides as necessary, until the mixture is creamy and smooth.
4. Place the mousse in glasses or serving dishes.
5. To help it set, refrigerate for at least 30 minutes.
6. Add fresh berries, chopped almonds, or shredded coconut as a garnish when it's time to serve.
7. Enjoy this decadent, creamy chocolate mousse without feeling guilty.

2. Nutcracker Energy Bites

Ingredients:
1/2 cup nut butter (such as almond or peanut butter) and 1 cup rolled oats.
  - 1/4 cup pure maple syrup or honey
  - 1/4 cup finely chopped nuts, such as cashews, almonds, or walnuts
  - 1/4 cup dried fruit, such as raisins or chopped dates
  - 14 cup optional micro chocolate chips
  – One teaspoon of vanilla extract
  – A dash of salt

- Directions: 1. Combine all the ingredients in a mixing bowl.

   2. Stir the mixture until it is fully incorporated and stays together.

   3. Using your hands, form the mixture into tiny bite-sized balls.

   4. Set the energy bites on a parchment-lined baking sheet.

   5. To help them set up, put them in the fridge for at least 30 minutes.

   6. Place the energy bites in the fridge in an airtight container.

   7. Have one or two on hand every time you want a quick and wholesome snack.

3. Baked Apple Chips

Ingredients:
2 apples (such as Honeycrisp or Granny Smith), 1 teaspoon cinnamon.

- **Requirements:**
   1. Set the oven temperature to 225°F (110°C).
   2. After removing the cores, finely slice the apples.
   3. Place the apple slices on a parchment-lined baking sheet in a single layer.
   4. Evenly sprinkling cinnamon over the apple pieces.
   5. Bake for 1 to 1.5 hours in a preheated oven, turning the slices over halfway.

6. When the apple slices are crisp and golden brown, remove from the oven.

7. Allow them to cool completely before consuming these naturally crunchy and sweet delicacies.

You may indulge in sweet desires while adding healthy ingredients with these guilt-free treats. These sweets, which range from the velvety avocado mousse to the nutty energy nibbles and crunchy baked apple chips, are made to be savored guilt-free. Enjoy each guilt-free bite while embracing the delight of healthy desserts and indulgences.

-Decadent Dairy-Free Delights

For those who follow a dairy-free lifestyle or have lactose intolerance, it can be challenging to find indulgent desserts that still deliver on taste and texture. This chapter presents a collection of luscious and satisfying dairy-free desserts that will leave you feeling completely indulged. Let's dive into the realm of dairy-free delights and discover the joy of guilt-free indulgence.

1. Rich Chocolate Coconut Pudding
- **Ingredients:**
  - 1 can full-fat coconut milk
  - 1/4 cup cocoa powder

- 1/4 cup pure maple syrup or other sweetener of choice
- 2 tablespoons cornstarch
- 1 teaspoon vanilla extract
- Pinch of salt
- Optional toppings: shredded coconut, fresh berries, or chopped nuts

- **Instructions:**

1. In a saucepan, whisk together the coconut milk, cocoa powder, maple syrup, cornstarch, vanilla extract, and salt.

2. Place the saucepan over medium heat and bring the mixture to a gentle simmer, whisking constantly.

3. Continue to cook and whisk until the mixture thickens to a pudding-like consistency, about 5-7 minutes.

4. Remove the saucepan from heat and let the pudding cool slightly.

5. Transfer the pudding into serving dishes or glasses and refrigerate for at least 2 hours or until set.

6. Serve chilled, topped with shredded coconut, fresh berries, or chopped nuts if desired.

7. Indulge in the creamy and rich goodness of this dairy-free chocolate pudding.

2. Velvety Cashew Cheesecake

- **Ingredients for the crust:**
- 1 1/2 cups almond flour

- 1/4 cup coconut oil, melted
- 2 tablespoons pure maple syrup

- Ingredients for the filling:
- 2 cups raw cashews, soaked in water for at least 4 hours or overnight
- 1/2 cup full-fat coconut milk
- 1/4 cup lemon juice
- 1/4 cup pure maple syrup
- 1/4 cup coconut oil, melted
- 1 teaspoon vanilla extract
- Pinch of salt

- Instructions:
1. In a mixing bowl, combine the almond flour, melted coconut oil, and maple syrup for the crust. Mix until well combined.
2. Press the crust mixture evenly into the bottom of a springform pan or individual tart pans.
3. In a blender or food processor, combine the soaked cashews, coconut milk, lemon juice, maple syrup, melted coconut oil, vanilla extract, and salt. Blend until smooth and creamy.
4. Pour the cashew filling over the prepared crust and smooth the top with a spatula.
5. Place the cheesecake in the refrigerator and let it chill for at least 4 hours or overnight until set.
6. Before serving, remove the cheesecake from the pan and slice into desired portions.
7. Enjoy the velvety texture and delightful flavors of this dairy-free cashew cheesecake.

3. Creamy Coconut Chia Pudding

- **Ingredients:**
  - 1 can full-fat coconut milk
  - 1/4 cup chia seeds
  - 2 tablespoons pure maple syrup or other sweetener of choice
  - 1 teaspoon vanilla extract
  - Optional toppings: fresh berries, sliced banana, toasted coconut flakes

- **Instructions:**
  1. In a bowl, whisk together the coconut milk, chia seeds, maple syrup, and vanilla extract.
  2. Let the mixture sit for about 10 minutes, then whisk again to prevent clumping.
  3. Cover the bowl and refrigerate for at least 2 hours or overnight until the chia seeds have absorbed the liquid and thickened the pudding.
  4. Stir the pudding before serving and adjust the sweetness if desired.
  5. Divide the pudding into serving dishes and top with fresh berries, sliced banana, or toasted coconut flakes.
  6. Enjoy the creamy and nutritious goodness of this dairy-free coconut chia pudding.

These decadent dairy-free delights offer a world of indulgence for those who embrace a dairy-free lifestyle. From the rich chocolate coconut pudding to the velvety cashew cheesecake and creamy coconut chia pudding, these desserts prove that dairy-free can still be utterly satisfying. Embrace the flavors and textures of these guilt-free indulgences and savor each delightful bite.

- Baked Goodness for the Sweet Tooth

Indulging in freshly baked treats is a delightful way to satisfy cravings and enjoy a moment of pure bliss. This chapter presents a collection of mouthwatering recipes for baked goods that are sure to delight your taste buds. From classic favorites to innovative creations, let's explore the realm of baked goodness and embark on a sweet journey.

1. Classic Chocolate Chip Cookies

- **Ingredients:**
  - 1 cup dairy-free butter, softened
  - 1 cup granulated sugar
  - 1 cup brown sugar, packed
  - 2 teaspoons vanilla extract
  - 2 flaxseed eggs (2 tablespoons ground flaxseed + 6 tablespoons water)
  - 3 cups all-purpose flour
  - 1 teaspoon baking soda

- 1/2 teaspoon salt
- 1 1/2 cups dairy-free chocolate chips

- **Instructions:**
1. Preheat the oven to 375°F (190°C) and line a baking sheet with parchment paper.
2. In a mixing bowl, cream together the dairy-free butter, granulated sugar, and brown sugar until light and fluffy.
3. Add the vanilla extract and flaxseed eggs, and mix until well combined.
4. In a separate bowl, whisk together the flour, baking soda, and salt.
5. Gradually add the dry ingredients to the wet ingredients, mixing until just combined.
6. Fold in the dairy-free chocolate chips.
7. Drop rounded tablespoonfuls of dough onto the prepared baking sheet, spacing them about 2 inches apart.
8. Bake for 10-12 minutes or until the edges are golden brown.
9. Remove from the oven and let the cookies cool on the baking sheet for a few minutes before transferring them to a wire rack to cool completely.
10. Enjoy these classic chocolate chip cookies with a glass of dairy-free milk for the ultimate treat.

2. Cinnamon Swirl Banana Bread

- **Ingredients:**
  - 3 ripe bananas, mashed
  - 1/2 cup coconut sugar or brown sugar
  - 1/4 cup dairy-free butter, melted
  - 1 flaxseed egg (1 tablespoon ground flaxseed + 3 tablespoons water)
  - 1 teaspoon vanilla extract
  - 1 1/2 cups all-purpose flour
  - 1 teaspoon baking soda
  - 1/2 teaspoon salt
  - 1 teaspoon ground cinnamon
  - 1/4 cup dairy-free milk
  - For the cinnamon swirl:
    - 1/4 cup coconut sugar or brown sugar
    - 1 tablespoon ground cinnamon

- **Instructions:**
  1. Preheat the oven to 350°F (175°C) and grease a loaf pan.
  2. In a large mixing bowl, combine the mashed bananas, coconut sugar, melted dairy-free butter, flaxseed egg, and vanilla extract.
  3. In a separate bowl, whisk together the flour, baking soda, salt, and ground cinnamon.

4. Gradually add the dry ingredients to the banana mixture, alternating with the dairy-free milk, and mix until just combined.

5. In a small bowl, mix together the coconut sugar and ground cinnamon for the cinnamon swirl.

6. Pour half of the banana bread batter into the prepared loaf pan.

7. Sprinkle half of the cinnamon sugar mixture over the batter.

8. Pour the remaining batter on top, followed by the remaining cinnamon sugar mixture.

9. Use a knife to swirl the cinnamon sugar mixture into the batter.

10. Bake for 50-60 minutes or until a toothpick inserted into the center comes out clean.

11. Allow the banana bread to cool in the pan for 10 minutes before transferring it to a wire rack to cool completely.

12. Slice and savor the delectable cinnamon swirl banana bread with a warm cup of tea or coffee.

3. Vanilla Bean Cupcakes with Dairy-Free Buttercream Frosting

- Ingredients for the cupcakes:
  - 1 1/2 cups all-purpose flour
  - 1 1/2 teaspoons baking powder
  - 1/4 teaspoon salt

- 1/2 cup dairy-free butter, softened
- 1 cup granulated sugar
- 2 flaxseed eggs (2 tablespoons ground flaxseed + 6 tablespoons water)
- 1 teaspoon vanilla extract
- 3/4 cup dairy-free milk

- Ingredients for the buttercream frosting:
- 1 cup dairy-free butter, softened
- 4 cups powdered sugar
- 2-3 tablespoons dairy-free milk
- 1 teaspoon vanilla extract

- Instructions for the cupcakes:
1. Preheat the oven to 350°F (175°C) and line a cupcake tin with paper liners.
2. In a medium bowl, whisk together the flour, baking powder, and salt.
3. In a separate bowl, cream together the dairy-free butter and granulated sugar until light and fluffy.
4. Add the flaxseed eggs and vanilla extract, and mix until well combined.
5. Gradually add the dry ingredients to the butter mixture, alternating with the dairy-free milk, and mix until just combined.
6. Fill each cupcake liner about two-thirds full with the batter.
7. Bake for 18-20 minutes or until a toothpick inserted into the center of a cupcake comes out clean.

8. Remove from the oven and let the cupcakes cool in the tin for a few minutes before transferring them to a wire rack to cool completely.

- Instructions for the buttercream frosting:
1. In a mixing bowl, beat the dairy-free butter until creamy.
2. Gradually add the powdered sugar, one cup at a time, and mix until smooth and fluffy.
3. Add the dairy-free milk and vanilla extract, and continue to beat until well combined and creamy.
4. Once the cupcakes have cooled completely, frost them with the dairy-free buttercream frosting using a piping bag or spatula.
5. Decorate with sprinkles or other toppings if desired.
6. Indulge in these heavenly vanilla bean cupcakes with dairy-free buttercream frosting for a delightful and sweet treat.

These recipes for baked goodness will satisfy your sweet tooth without compromising on taste or dietary preferences. Whether you're craving classic chocolate chip cookies, a cinnamon-infused banana bread, or vanilla bean cupcakes with dairy-free buttercream frosting, these recipes will bring joy to your taste buds. Enjoy the aromas and flavors of freshly baked treats that are sure to delight both you and your loved ones.

- Refreshing Frozen Treats

These recipes are not only delicious but also made with wholesome ingredients to ensure you're nourishing your body while enjoying a frozen delight. From fruity popsicles to creamy ice creams, let's dive into the world of refreshing frozen treats and discover your new favorites.

1. Berry Blast Popsicles

- Ingredients:
 - 2 cups mixed berries (strawberries, blueberries, raspberries)
 - 1/4 cup maple syrup or honey
 - 1 cup coconut water
 - 1 tablespoon fresh lemon juice

- Instructions:
 1. In a blender, combine the mixed berries, maple syrup or honey, coconut water, and lemon juice.
 2. Blend until smooth and well combined.
 3. Pour the mixture into popsicle molds, leaving a little space at the top for expansion.
 4. Insert popsicle sticks into each mold.
 5. Place the molds in the freezer and freeze for at least 4 hours or until completely solid.

6. To remove the popsicles from the molds, run warm water over the molds for a few seconds and gently pull the popsicles out.

7. Enjoy the refreshing and fruity goodness of these homemade Berry Blast Popsicles.

2. Creamy Coconut Mango Sorbet

- **Ingredients:**
  - 2 ripe mangoes, peeled and diced
  - 1 can full-fat coconut milk
  - 1/4 cup maple syrup or honey
  - 1 tablespoon fresh lime juice

- **Instructions**:

1. Place the diced mangoes in a blender or food processor.

2. Add the coconut milk, maple syrup or honey, and lime juice.

3. Blend until smooth and creamy.

4. Pour the mixture into a shallow dish or ice cream maker.

5. If using a dish, cover it with plastic wrap and place it in the freezer.

6. Every hour, remove the dish from the freezer and stir the mixture to break up any ice crystals.

7. Repeat this process for about 4-6 hours or until the sorbet reaches the desired consistency.

8. Serve the creamy coconut mango sorbet in bowls or cones and savor the tropical flavors.

3. Vegan Chocolate Nice Cream

- **Ingredients:**
  - 4 ripe bananas, peeled and frozen
  - 1/4 cup unsweetened cocoa powder
  - 2 tablespoons maple syrup or agave nectar
  - 1/2 teaspoon vanilla extract

- **Instructions:**
  1. Place the frozen bananas, cocoa powder, maple syrup or agave nectar, and vanilla extract in a blender or food processor.
  2. Blend until the mixture is smooth and creamy, resembling soft-serve ice cream.
  3. You may need to stop and scrape down the sides of the blender or food processor a few times to ensure everything is well combined.
  4. Transfer the nice cream to a container and freeze for an additional 1-2 hours to firm up.
  5. Serve the vegan chocolate nice cream in bowls or cones, and indulge in the guilt-free pleasure of this creamy and chocolaty frozen treat.

4. Watermelon Lime Granita

- Ingredients:
  - 4 cups cubed seedless watermelon
  - 2 tablespoons fresh lime juice
  - 2 tablespoons honey or agave nectar

- Instructions:
  1. Place the watermelon cubes, lime juice, and honey or agave nectar in a blender or food processor.
  2. Blend until smooth and well combined.
  3. Pour the mixture into a shallow dish.
  4. Place the dish in the freezer and let it freeze for about 1 hour.
  5. Using a fork, scrape the frozen mixture to create fluffy ice crystals.
  6. Return the dish to the freezer and repeat the scraping process every 30 minutes for about 2-3 hours or until the entire mixture is transformed into granita.
  7. Serve the watermelon lime granita in bowls or glasses, and enjoy the refreshing and icy texture of this delightful frozen treat.

5. Mint Chocolate Chip Ice Cream Sandwiches

- Ingredients:
  - 2 cups raw cashews, soaked for 4-6 hours and drained

- 1 cup coconut milk
- 1/4 cup maple syrup or agave nectar
- 1 teaspoon vanilla extract
- 1/2 teaspoon peppermint extract
- 1/4 cup dark chocolate chips
- 20 small vegan chocolate cookies

- **Instructions:**
1. In a blender or food processor, combine the soaked cashews, coconut milk, maple syrup or agave nectar, vanilla extract, and peppermint extract.
2. Blend until smooth and creamy.
3. Stir in the dark chocolate chips.
4. Transfer the mixture to a container and freeze for about 2 hours or until firm.
5. Take 1 tablespoon of the mixture and place it between two vegan chocolate cookies to form a sandwich.
6. Repeat with the remaining mixture and cookies.
7. Return the sandwiches to the freezer for an additional 1-2 hours to set.
8. Enjoy these mint chocolate chip ice cream sandwiches as a satisfying and refreshing frozen treat.

These refreshing frozen treats offer a variety of flavors and textures to satisfy your cravings for cool and delicious desserts. Whether you prefer fruity popsicles, creamy sorbets, or indulgent nice creams, these recipes provide a range of options to please your taste buds. Enjoy these frozen delights and treat yourself to a refreshing and delightful experience.

Chapter 9: Hydration and Nourishment for Optimal Breastfeeding

- Quenching Infused Water Recipes

In Chapter 9 of our cookbook, we explore the importance of hydration and nourishment for optimal breastfeeding. Staying hydrated is crucial for maintaining milk production and overall well-being during this special phase of motherhood. To make hydrating more enjoyable and flavorful, we've gathered a collection of quenching infused water recipes that will not only keep you hydrated but also infuse your water with a burst of refreshing flavors and beneficial nutrients. Let's dive into the world of infused waters and discover delicious combinations to support your breastfeeding journey.

1. Citrus Mint Refresher

- Ingredients:
- 1 lemon, sliced
- 1 lime, sliced
- 1 orange, sliced
- A handful of fresh mint leaves

- 4 cups of filtered water
- Ice cubes (optional)

- Instructions:
   1. Place the lemon slices, lime slices, orange slices, and fresh mint leaves in a pitcher.
   2. Fill the pitcher with 4 cups of filtered water.
   3. Stir gently to combine the ingredients.
   4. If desired, add ice cubes to the pitcher to keep the water cool.
   5. Let the infused water sit in the refrigerator for at least 1 hour to allow the flavors to meld.
   6. Pour the refreshing Citrus Mint Refresher into glasses, garnish with additional mint leaves if desired, and enjoy the zesty and invigorating flavors.

2. Berry Blast Infusion

- Ingredients:
   - 1 cup fresh strawberries, hulled and halved
   - 1 cup fresh blueberries
   - 1 cup fresh raspberries
   - 4 cups of filtered water
   - Ice cubes (optional)

- Instructions:
   1. In a pitcher, combine the strawberries, blueberries, and raspberries.
   2. Add 4 cups of filtered water to the pitcher.

3. Stir gently to mix the berries and water.

4. If desired, add ice cubes to the pitcher for a chilled infusion.

5. Allow the Berry Blast Infusion to sit in the refrigerator for at least 1 hour to infuse the water with the vibrant flavors of the berries.

6. Pour the fruity and refreshing infusion into glasses, and savor the sweet and tangy notes of the berries.

3. Cucumber and Mint Elixir

- Ingredients:
- 1 cucumber, thinly sliced
- A handful of fresh mint leaves
- 4 cups of filtered water
- Ice cubes (optional)

- Instructions:

1. Place the cucumber slices and fresh mint leaves in a pitcher.

2. Pour 4 cups of filtered water into the pitcher.

3. Stir gently to combine the ingredients.

4. If desired, add ice cubes to the pitcher to keep the water cool.

5. Let the Cucumber and Mint Elixir infuse in the refrigerator for at least 1 hour to release the refreshing flavors.

6. Pour the revitalizing elixir into glasses, and enjoy the crisp and rejuvenating taste of cucumber and mint.

4. Tropical Pineapple and Coconut Water Blend

- Ingredients:
  - 2 cups fresh pineapple chunks
  - 4 cups coconut water
  - Ice cubes (optional)

- Instructions:
  1. In a blender, combine the fresh pineapple chunks and coconut water.
  2. Blend until smooth and well combined.
  3. If desired, add ice cubes to a glass before pouring in the pineapple and coconut water blend for a chilled treat.
  4. Savor the tropical

 flavors of the Pineapple and Coconut Water Blend while reaping the hydrating benefits of coconut water.

5. Watermelon and Basil Infusion

- Ingredients:
  - 2 cups cubed seedless watermelon
  - A handful of fresh basil leaves
  - 4 cups of filtered water

- Ice cubes (optional)

- **Instructions:**
   1. In a pitcher, combine the cubed watermelon and fresh basil leaves.
   2. Pour 4 cups of filtered water into the pitcher.
   3. Stir gently to mix the watermelon and basil with the water.
   4. If desired, add ice cubes to the pitcher for a chilled infusion.
   5. Allow the Watermelon and Basil Infusion to sit in the refrigerator for at least 1 hour to infuse the water with the refreshing flavors of watermelon and the aromatic essence of basil.
   6. Pour the infused water into glasses, and relish the light and refreshing taste of this delightful combination.

These quenching infused water recipes provide a flavorful and hydrating way to support your breastfeeding journey. By infusing your water with the natural flavors of citrus fruits, berries, cucumbers, and herbs, you can elevate your hydration routine and enjoy the benefits of these nourishing ingredients. Stay refreshed, replenished, and energized with these delightful infused water creations as you embrace the journey of breastfeeding and motherhood.

- Replenishing Smoothies and Mocktails

These refreshing and nutritious beverages are designed to replenish your energy, provide essential nutrients, and offer a delightful way to stay hydrated. Whether you're in need of a quick pick-me-up or a flavorful mocktail to enjoy during a special occasion, this chapter has you covered. Let's dive into the world of replenishing smoothies and mocktails and discover a variety of delicious recipes to nourish and indulge in.

1. Berry Burst Smoothie

- Ingredients:
 - 1 cup mixed berries (such as strawberries, blueberries, and raspberries)
   - 1 ripe banana
   - 1 cup almond milk (or any milk of your choice)
   - 1 tablespoon chia seeds
   - 1 tablespoon honey or maple syrup (optional)
   - Ice cubes (optional)

- Instructions:
   1. In a blender, combine the mixed berries, ripe banana, almond milk, chia seeds, and sweetener if desired.
   2. Blend until smooth and creamy.

3. If desired, add ice cubes to the blender for a chilled smoothie.

4. Pour the Berry Burst Smoothie into a glass and enjoy the vibrant flavors and antioxidant-rich goodness.

2. Green Goddess Smoothie

- Ingredients:
  - 1 ripe avocado
  - 1 ripe banana
  - Handful of spinach leaves
  - 1 cup coconut water
  - 1 tablespoon almond butter
  - 1 tablespoon honey or agave syrup (optional)
  - Ice cubes (optional)

- Instructions:

1. In a blender, combine the ripe avocado, ripe banana, spinach leaves, coconut water, almond butter, and sweetener if desired.

2. Blend until smooth and creamy.

3. If desired, add ice cubes to the blender for a chilled smoothie.

4. Pour the Green Goddess Smoothie into a glass and enjoy the nourishing blend of creamy avocado, nutrient-rich spinach, and refreshing coconut water.

3. Tropical Mocktail

- Ingredients:
  - 1 cup pineapple juice
  - 1/2 cup orange juice
  - 1/2 cup coconut water
  - 1 tablespoon lime juice
  - Splash of sparkling water or soda (optional)
  - Pineapple wedge or mint sprig for garnish (optional)
  - Ice cubes

- Instructions:
  1. In a shaker or pitcher, combine the pineapple juice, orange juice, coconut water, and lime juice.
  2. Shake or stir well to mix the flavors.
  3. If desired, add a splash of sparkling water or soda for a fizzy twist.
  4. Fill a glass with ice cubes and pour the Tropical Mocktail over the ice.
  5. Garnish with a pineapple wedge or mint sprig, if desired.
  6. Sip and enjoy the tropical flavors of this refreshing mocktail.

4. Energizing Matcha Smoothie

- Ingredients:
  - 1 teaspoon matcha powder
  - 1 ripe banana

- 1 cup almond milk (or any milk of your choice)
- 1 tablespoon honey or agave syrup
- 1/2 teaspoon vanilla extract
- Handful of baby spinach leaves
- Ice cubes (optional)

- **Instructions:**
1. In a blender, combine the matcha powder, ripe banana, almond milk, sweetener, vanilla extract, and baby spinach leaves.
2. Blend until smooth and creamy.
3. If desired, add ice cubes to the blender for a chilled smoothie.
4. Pour the Energizing Matcha Smoothie into a glass and savor the vibrant green color and the energizing boost of matcha.

5. Mocktail Mule

- **Ingredients:**
  - 1/2 cup ginger beer
  - 1/4 cup lime juice
  - 1/4 cup sparkling water
  - 1 tablespoon honey or agave syrup (optional)
  - Sliced lime for garnish (optional)
  - Ice cubes

- **Instructions:**

1. In a glass, combine the ginger beer, lime juice, sparkling water, and sweetener if desired.

2. Stir well to mix the flavors.

3. Fill the glass with ice cubes.

4. Garnish with a slice of lime, if desired.

5. Sip and enjoy the refreshing and tangy flavors of the Mocktail Mule.

These replenishing smoothies and mocktails are not only delicious but also provide essential nutrients to support your well-being during the breastfeeding journey. Whether you're seeking a boost of antioxidants, a refreshing tropical blend, or a vibrant green energy drink, this chapter offers a variety of options to satisfy your cravings and replenish your body. Enjoy these delightful beverages as a nourishing treat or share them with friends and family during special occasions. Cheers to nourishment and hydration!

- Herbal Teas for Milk Production

For millennia, breastfeeding moms have utilized herbal teas to enhance lactation and encourage healthy milk production. These teas provide a calming and delectable method to nourish your body and improve your breastfeeding journey. They are packed with natural ingredients and medicinal herbs. Join us as we investigate a selection of herbal teas designed expressly to promote milk production and to offer solace and relaxation.

Tea with Fenugreek

Ingredients:
- 1 tea bag of fenugreek or 1 teaspoon of dried fenugreek leaves
  – One cup of hot water
  - Lemon or honey, optional

- **Requirements:**
  1. Put the fenugreek tea bag or dried leaves in a cup.
  2. Cover the fenugreek with hot water.
  3. To extract the tastes and health benefits, let it steep for 5 to 10 minutes.
  4. For more flavor, if preferred, add honey or lemon.
  5. Stir the fenugreek tea thoroughly before drinking it to enjoy its nutty and earthy flavor while promoting milk production.

Blessed Thistle Tea

Ingredients:
1 tea bag of blessed thistle or 1 teaspoon of dried blessed thistle leaves
  – One cup of hot water
  - Optional honey or cinnamon

- Requirements:

1. Fill a cup with tea made from blessed thistle leaves or dried blessed thistle leaves.

2. Cover the blessed thistle with hot water.

3. Permit the mixture to steep for 5 to 10 minutes to draw out the tastes and therapeutic benefits.

4. For more sweetness and warmth, if preferred, add honey or a dash of cinnamon.

5. Stir thoroughly and enjoy Blessed Thistle Tea's distinct and slightly bitter flavor, which is renowned for its ability to increase milk production.

Fennel seed tea

Ingredients

- One teaspoon of fennel seeds or one fennel tea bag
- One cup of hot water
- Optional honey or ginger

- Requirements:

1. Use a mortar and pestle to slightly crush the fennel seeds.

2. Add the fennel tea bag or crushed fennel seeds to a cup.

3. Cover the fennel with hot water.

4. Allow it to steep for 5 to 10 minutes to release the flavorful aromas and therapeutic properties.

5. You can add honey or a slice of ginger for a little warmth and sweetness, if you like.

6. Stir thoroughly and savor the calming, anise-like flavor of fennel seed tea, which is renowned for increasing milk production.

Raspberry Leaf Tea

Ingredients
- 1 teaspoon dried raspberry leaves or 1 raspberry leaf tea bag
  – One cup of hot water
  - Lemon or honey, optional

- **Requirements:**
1. Put the raspberry leaf tea bag or dried raspberry leaves in a cup.
2. Cover the raspberry leaves with hot water.
3. Let it steep for 5 to 10 minutes to let the flavors and health benefits permeate the water.
4. For a hint of sweetness or tanginess, if preferred, add honey or a squeeze of lemon.
5. Give Raspberry Leaf Tea a good stir and savor its herbal, slightly earthy flavor. Raspberry Leaf Tea is renowned for its nourishing properties for the female reproductive system and milk production.

5. Tea made from nettles

Ingredients:
1 teaspoon dried nettle leaves or 1 tea bag of nettle leaves
   - 1 cup hot water with optional honey or mint

- **Requirements:**
   1. Fill a cup with dried nettle leaves or nettle leaf tea.
   2. Cover the nettle leaves with hot water.
   3. Allow it to steep for 5 to 10 minutes to draw out the flavors and therapeutic qualities.
   4. For more sweetness or a cool touch, if desired, add honey or a sprig of fresh mint.
   5. Stir well and savor the grassy, somewhat herbal flavor of nettle leaf tea, which has been shown to increase milk production and has a high vitamin content.

During your nursing journey, these herbal teas provide a relaxing and natural method to assist your milk production. Take a time to relax while you sip on these healthful and aromatic beverages, whether you prefer them warm or chilled. One cup at a time, embrace the strength of herbs and their ability to improve your breastfeeding experience.

-Nutrient-Packed Hydration Tips

Let us explore the importance of hydration for breastfeeding moms and provide you with nutrient-packed hydration tips. Staying properly hydrated is essential for maintaining your milk supply, supporting your overall health, and ensuring optimal breastfeeding success. We'll guide you through various hydration strategies and share tips on incorporating nutrient-rich beverages into your daily routine. Let's dive into the world of hydration and discover ways to nourish your body with refreshing and beneficial drinks.

1. Infused Water

- Add slices of fresh fruits like lemon, lime, strawberries, or cucumber to a pitcher of water.
- Let it sit for a few hours or overnight to infuse the water with natural flavors.
- Sip on this refreshing infused water throughout the day to stay hydrated and enjoy a hint of fruity goodness.

2. Herbal Iced Tea

- Brew a pot of herbal tea using flavors like chamomile, peppermint, hibiscus, or rooibos.
- Allow the tea to cool and refrigerate it.
- Serve over ice for a refreshing and hydrating herbal iced tea, packed with antioxidants and beneficial plant compounds.

3. Coconut Water

- Enjoy the natural electrolyte-rich goodness of coconut water, which helps replenish minerals lost during breastfeeding.
- Drink it chilled or use it as a base for refreshing smoothies and mocktails.

4. Fresh Fruit Smoothies

- Blend together a variety of fresh fruits, such as berries, bananas, mangoes, or pineapple, with a liquid of your choice, such as almond milk or coconut water.

- Add in a handful of spinach or kale for an extra nutrient boost.
- Sip on these delicious and hydrating fruit smoothies, which provide essential vitamins and minerals.

5. Homemade Electrolyte Drinks

- Create your own electrolyte drink by mixing coconut water, a pinch of sea salt, a squeeze of lemon or lime juice, and a natural sweetener like honey or maple syrup.
- This homemade electrolyte drink helps replenish electrolytes and keeps you hydrated, especially during hot days or periods of increased physical activity.

Remember, staying hydrated is crucial for your well-being and milk production. Incorporate these nutrient-packed hydration tips into your daily routine to ensure you're providing your body with the necessary fluids and nourishment. Hydrate with intention, and enjoy the refreshing and beneficial beverages that support your breastfeeding journey. Cheers to health and hydration!

Chapter 10: Self-Care and Wellness for Breastfeeding Moms

- Mindful Eating Practices

This chapter focuses on the concept of mindful eating practices and how they can contribute to your overall well-being as you navigate the beautiful and demanding journey of breastfeeding. We explore the transformative power of being present in the moment, making conscious food choices, and nourishing your body with intention. Let's embark on a journey of self-care and discover how mindful eating practices can support you on this incredible adventure.

1. Understanding Mindful Eating

- Learn about the principles of mindful eating, which involve being fully present and engaged in the act of eating.
- Discover how to listen to your body's hunger and fullness cues, and cultivate a deeper connection with your body's nutritional needs.

- Explore techniques such as mindful breathing, mindful chewing, and savoring the flavors and textures of your food.

2. Cultivating Food Awareness

- Develop a heightened sense of awareness around the food you consume and its impact on your well-being.
- Explore the nutritional benefits of different foods and how they can support your energy levels, milk production, and overall health.
- Become mindful of the connection between the food you eat and the nourishment it provides to both you and your baby.

3. Building a Nourishing Plate

- Learn how to create balanced and nourishing meals by incorporating a variety of food groups.
- Explore the importance of whole grains, lean proteins, healthy fats, and a rainbow of fruits and vegetables in supporting your nutritional needs.
- Discover creative ways to make your meals visually appealing, satisfying to the palate, and packed with nutrients.

4. Mindful Eating Rituals

- Establish rituals around mealtimes to create a sense of calm and intention.

- Set aside dedicated time for meals, free from distractions, to fully engage with your food and enjoy the sensory experience.
- Practice gratitude for the nourishment you receive and foster a positive mindset towards the food you consume.

5. Self-Care Practices

- Prioritize self-care as an integral part of your breastfeeding journey.
- Explore activities that bring you joy, relaxation, and rejuvenation.
- Engage in gentle exercise, meditation, journaling, or other self-care practices that help you recharge and nurture your mind, body, and soul.

By embracing mindful eating practices and incorporating self-care into your daily routine, you can enhance your overall well-being as a breastfeeding mom. Nourishing yourself with intention and cultivating a positive relationship with food can have a profound impact on your physical health, emotional well-being, and milk production. Use this chapter as a guide to explore the transformative power of mindful eating and self-care, and discover how they can contribute to a more fulfilling and balanced breastfeeding experience.

- Balancing Nutrition and Rest

As a new mother, it's crucial to nourish your body with the right nutrients while also ensuring you get the rest you need to support your overall health and milk production. This chapter focuses on practical strategies for maintaining a well-rounded diet and prioritizing adequate rest, allowing you to optimize your breastfeeding journey and care for yourself in the process. Let's delve into the art of balancing nutrition and rest and discover ways to create harmony in your daily life.

1. Prioritizing Nutrient-Dense Foods

- Learn about the key nutrients necessary for breastfeeding moms, such as protein, healthy fats, vitamins, and minerals.
- Explore a variety of nutrient-dense foods that can support your energy levels, milk supply, and postpartum recovery.
- Discover delicious recipes that incorporate these nutrients and provide a well-rounded, nourishing diet.

2. Meal Planning and Preparation

- Discover the benefits of meal planning and preparation for maintaining a healthy diet as a busy breastfeeding mom.
- Learn practical tips for efficient meal planning, including batch cooking, utilizing leftovers, and incorporating convenience foods without compromising nutrition.
- Create a meal plan that incorporates a balance of macronutrients and a variety of colorful fruits, vegetables, whole grains, and lean proteins.

3. Snacking for Sustained Energy

- Explore the importance of healthy snacks in maintaining energy levels and supporting milk production.
- Discover wholesome snack ideas that are easy to prepare and provide a combination of protein, fiber, and healthy fats.
- Learn how to choose snacks that keep you satiated and provide a sustained release of energy throughout the day.

4. Adequate Rest and Recovery

- Understand the significance of rest and recovery in promoting overall health and well-being.
- Learn strategies for prioritizing rest, including setting boundaries, establishing a sleep routine, and seeking support from loved ones.

- Discover relaxation techniques and self-care practices that can help you recharge and rejuvenate during the demanding breastfeeding phase.

5. Finding Balance and Flexibility

- Recognize that finding balance as a breastfeeding mom involves embracing flexibility and being kind to yourself.
- Understand that each day may bring different challenges and priorities, and adapt your nutrition and rest practices accordingly.
- Learn to listen to your body's cues and make adjustments as needed to maintain a sustainable and nourishing lifestyle.

By focusing on balancing nutrition and rest, you can optimize your health, milk production, and overall well-being as a breastfeeding mom. Prioritizing nutrient-dense foods, efficient meal planning, and adequate rest allows you to nurture yourself while caring for your little one. Use this chapter as a guide to find harmony in your daily life, and embrace the journey of nourishing both your body and your baby with love, care, and balance.

- Postpartum Nutrition for Recovery

The postpartum period is a time of immense physical and emotional changes, and nourishing your body with the right nutrients is essential for your healing, energy levels, and overall well-being. This chapter focuses on providing comprehensive guidance on postpartum nutrition, offering practical tips, delicious recipes, and valuable information to support your recovery journey. Let's explore the importance of postpartum nutrition and discover ways to nourish your body during this special time.

1. Understanding Postpartum Nutrition

- Learn about the unique nutritional needs during the postpartum period, including increased energy requirements and specific nutrient considerations.
- Explore the importance of replenishing nutrients lost during childbirth and supporting your body's healing processes.
- Understand how nutrition can impact breastfeeding, mood, energy levels, and overall postpartum recovery.

2. Key Nutrients for Postpartum Healing

- Discover the essential nutrients for postpartum recovery, such as protein, iron, calcium, omega-3 fatty acids, and vitamin C.
- Learn about food sources that are rich in these nutrients and how to incorporate them into your meals.
- Explore the benefits of consuming nutrient-dense foods to support tissue repair, hormone balance, and optimal recovery.

3. Building a Nourishing Postpartum Plate

- Explore strategies for creating balanced and nourishing meals that incorporate a variety of food groups.
- Learn how to include foods that promote healing, such as lean proteins, whole grains, healthy fats, and plenty of fruits and vegetables.
- Discover simple and delicious recipes designed to support postpartum recovery while providing comfort and satisfaction.

4. Supporting Breastfeeding Through Nutrition

- Understand the connection between nutrition and breastfeeding, and how your dietary choices can impact milk production and quality.
- Learn about lactogenic foods that may enhance milk supply and explore ways to incorporate them into your meals and snacks.
- Discover the importance of hydration and tips for staying well-hydrated while breastfeeding.

- Recognize the significance of self-care and emotional well-being during the postpartum period.
- Explore the role of nutrition in supporting mental health and managing postpartum emotions.
- Discover recipes and practices that promote relaxation, stress reduction, and self-nurturing.

By focusing on postpartum nutrition for recovery, you can support your body's healing processes, replenish vital nutrients, and enhance your overall well-being during this transformative phase of motherhood. Use this chapter as a valuable resource to guide your postpartum nutrition journey, and embrace the opportunity to nourish and care for yourself as you embrace the joys and challenges of motherhood.

- Nurturing the Body and Mind

The journey of breastfeeding involves not only physical nourishment but also emotional well-being and self-care. This chapter focuses on holistic practices and strategies that promote the health and harmony of your body and mind. Let's delve into the art of nurturing the body and mind and discover ways to create a balanced and fulfilling breastfeeding experience.

1. The Mind-Body Connection

- Understand the powerful connection between the mind and body and how it influences your overall well-being.
- Explore the impact of stress, emotions, and mental health on breastfeeding and milk production.
- Learn techniques to cultivate mindfulness, presence, and positive thinking to support your overall health.

2. Self-Care Practices

- Prioritize self-care as an integral part of your breastfeeding journey.
- Explore activities that bring you joy, relaxation, and rejuvenation.
- Engage in gentle exercise, meditation, journaling, or other self-care practices that help you recharge and nurture your mind and body.

3. Emotional Well-being

- Acknowledge and address the range of emotions that may arise during the breastfeeding journey.
- Explore strategies for managing stress, anxiety, and postpartum mood changes.
- Seek support from loved ones, healthcare professionals, or support groups to nurture your emotional well-being.

4. Restorative Exercise

- Discover the benefits of gentle exercise for physical and mental well-being.

- Explore exercises that promote strength, flexibility, and relaxation.
- Find ways to incorporate exercise into your daily routine, considering your energy levels and time constraints.

5. Mindful Eating Practices

- Embrace the concept of mindful eating to foster a positive relationship with food.
- Learn to listen to your body's hunger and fullness cues and make conscious food choices.
- Practice gratitude for the nourishment you receive and savor the flavors and textures of your meals.

6. Connection and Support

- Recognize the importance of social connection and support during the breastfeeding journey.
- Seek out breastfeeding support groups, online communities, or lactation consultants who can provide guidance and encouragement.
- Share experiences and stories with other breastfeeding moms to foster a sense of community and camaraderie.

By nurturing both your body and mind, you can enhance your overall well-being and create a harmonious breastfeeding experience. Incorporating self-care practices, embracing positive thinking, and fostering emotional well-being can contribute to a more balanced and fulfilling journey. Use this chapter as a guide to explore the art of nurturing your body and mind, and celebrate the remarkable strength and resilience of motherhood.

Conclusion:

Embracing a Healthy and Joyful Breastfeeding Journey

In conclusion, "Eat to Latch" is not just a cookbook but a comprehensive guide to embracing a healthy and joyful breastfeeding journey. Throughout the chapters, we have explored various aspects of nutrition, self-care, and well-being that are essential for breastfeeding moms. We have delved into the understanding of nutritional needs, boosting milk supply, and enhancing milk quality through carefully selected ingredients and recipes.

From energizing smoothie bowls and protein-packed pancakes to vibrant salads, hearty grain bowls, and nourishing dinners for the whole family, we have provided a wide range of delicious and nutritious recipes to support your breastfeeding experience. We have also emphasized the importance of mindful eating, meal planning, and finding balance in your daily life to ensure you prioritize self-care and meet your nutritional needs.

Moreover, we have addressed the unique challenges and needs of breastfeeding moms, offering lactation-friendly recipes, postpartum nutrition for